Brenda McLeod

MW01518882

Because He Loved Me

Alexis Judy

WestBow
PRESS
A DIVISION OF THOMAS NELSON

Copyright © 2013 Alexis Judy.

All rights reserved. No part of this book may be used or reproduced by any means,
graphic, electronic, or mechanical, including photocopying, recording, taping or by any
information storage retrieval system without the written permission of the publisher
except in the case of brief quotations embodied in critical articles and reviews.

WestBow Press books may be ordered through booksellers or by contacting:

WestBow Press
A Division of Thomas Nelson
1663 Liberty Drive
Bloomington, IN 47403
www.westbowpress.com
1-(866) 928-1240

Because of the dynamic nature of the Internet, any web addresses or links contained in
this book may have changed since publication and may no longer be valid. The views
expressed in this work are solely those of the author and do not necessarily reflect the
views of the publisher, and the publisher hereby disclaims any responsibility for them.

Any people depicted in stock imagery provided by Thinkstock are models,
and such images are being used for illustrative purposes only.

Certain stock imagery © Thinkstock.

ISBN: 978-1-4497-8683-0 (e)
ISBN: 978-1-4497-8684-7 (sc)
ISBN: 978-1-4497-8685-4 (hc)

Library of Congress Control Number: 2013903852

Printed in the United States of America

WestBow Press rev. date: 3/20/2013

Hi there. My name's Alexis. I'm assuming you already know the gist of my story even though you haven't really dug in yet. If you don't know anything about me, you'll get there soon enough. I just want you to know that this book is telling a story in its most exposed, vulnerable, raw state. I've made the choice to leave it completely unedited because I feel that it will make the strongest impact that way. These writings were taken directly from my journal and put into this collection of memories just for you. Risky, I know. Will there be editorial mistakes and sentences that could flow better? Definitely. Yes, this book allows me to reminisce and reflect, but I want God to use this story to rock your world the same way it rocked mine. I hope that if nothing else, you see life from a new perspective and with deeper meaning. I pray that you're convicted, I long for you to be inspired, I hope that you find the one true hope, and I sincerely ask God that your heart is pierced with the power of authentic, radical, Jesus kind of love. And I hope you take that love and change this world with a story of your own.

Con Amor,

Lexi

The following pages consist of thin burgundy lines separating small white spaces containing the thoughts and emotions of a sixteen year old girl carrying the weight of the world. With magazine clippings and fancy adjectives I will put my heart on paper and my soul on wings.

Alexis Lee Judy

My Journey of Cancer Treatment

February First, Two-Thousand Ten

Dedications

<u>Mommy and Daddy</u> – The people responsible for making me the person I am today. And for that, I am forever grateful.

<u>My Sister (Caely)</u> – My wonderful, beautiful, best friend. You mean more than you know.

<u>My baby brothers (Harrison and Hayden)</u> – The two who keep me young and smiling. I love you.

<u>God</u> – The only one capable of pulling me through.

On January 8th, 2010, I was admitted to the oncology floor at The Children's Hospital of The King's Daughters.

On January 9th, 2010, I was officially diagnosed with Hodgkin's Lymphoma Cancer.

On January 17th, 2010, I turned 16 and ½.

I never imagined being in a hospital fighting cancer at 16 and ½.

I was forever changed.

Table of Contents

Wednesday, January 20th, 2010

    Sorry this took so long. So, The Children's Hospital of the King's Daughter's (CHKD) will give their patients a laptop with WIFI, but it won't access Facebook. Whackkk. So, I had to write all of this and save it on my email until now. I am finally home after 12 nights and 13 days in the hospital. Thank God. Oh, and just to let you know, it's gonna take you a while to read through this one.

    Hey guys. As most of you have already figured out, I have been diagnosed with Hodgkin's Lymphoma Cancer. Wow. Watching myself type that it's like I'm acting in a movie or something. That's how it's felt from the moment I heard those words. As I sit here on the hospital bed it's kind of hard not to ask myself, "What on earth are you doing here? You don't belong here." The response most people give me is usually something to the effect of, "Wow, you're kidding? You can't be serious. I don't believe it. It all came so fast and out of nowhere." My typical response is, "Ha, you're telling me."

All of this started back in November around Thanksgiving time. I had a terrible cough and nasty cold. Mom took me to the doctor, against my own will. I was determined I just had a common cold. Well, I was right. Or, for the time being anyways. The doctor told me she had seen a bunch of kids come in just like myself and she was sure it would go away in a couple of weeks. Well, a couple of weeks came and went and the cough was still there. So, I went back in. The doctor informed me that I either had walking pneumonia or bronchitis. Either way, it was the same treatment so she gave me the anti-biotic and an inhaler to help with the difficulty breathing. It improved, but it wasn't completely gone. I assumed there was still some pneumonia left down in my lungs, however, did not want to return to the doctor's office yet again. My mother and father didn't really care how I felt at this point, they knew I needed to go in. So, in again we went only to be diagnosed with another miscalculated guess. It was thought to be reoccurring asthma from when I was 8

(I had been diagnosed with exercise induced asthma, where the muscles around your lungs close in on your lungs whenever you exercise. At the time we were told children typically outgrow this by the age of twelve, which I did. It only lasted one soccer season. However, they are now discovering that more children are having it come back and therefore giving the reason my doctor assumed I had it.). So, she gave me an inhaler but just in case she also sent me for chest x-rays. I had basketball practice that night so I asked if it would be okay if I joined the team and she said, "Absolutely, that would actually be good for you." So, off I went to get the chest x-rays and then to the gym.

I went to basketball practice and ran my three laps without realizing just how close I came to death. I figured the medicine hadn't kicked in yet, or I didn't have enough. I finished up practice almost normally. After practice I wanted to go out to get pizza with some friends, but my dad wasn't all for the idea. Little did I know why. As I eventually headed out to the car with my sister because dad wouldn't answer my phone call and question to whether I could go or not, he ran into us. Quickly he grabbed my sister and I and walked us out to his truck where my two little brothers were already strapped in and as confused as we were. On our way out my coach said, "Alexis, what's going on?" and I told her I had "No clue." My dad was acting strange, double checking to make sure I had my coat on. I could tell he was talking to my mom and she was not acting like herself. They were both in a panic. My little brother started assuming things like the house was being robbed, that's what it sounded like. I had visions of her being held hostage but quickly ignored them when I realized how silly that sounded. I immediately began freaking out but the closer we got to the house the more frustrated I became because they wouldn't tell us anything. Within minutes we arrived at the house and dad went upstairs to check on my mom. My siblings and I just sat down stairs dazed and confused. Not long after, my dad came downstairs and told me that we had to go to the E.R. just to get checked out because they had the results of the chest x-rays I had taken that day. He just held me and I didn't bother fighting the tears.

We arrived at the E.R. and two of my uncles were there. I still didn't think too much of the situation, I just knew I had caring uncles. Eventually I was taken into a room so they could weigh me and check my vitals. Later on, I was taken back to a room to be checked out by a couple doctors who failed to inform me that their specialty was cancer because my parents didn't want me to know just yet. They wanted to be absolutely positive. So, I did a cat scan and blood work and all of those sorts of things I only pray I can forget, and then the doctor came back into the room to say the most life changing, ear piercing, heart stopping, un-imaginable, un-believable, words I have ever had to take in my lifetime. I remember it second by second,

"Alexis, do you know why you're here?"

"Umm, because they needed to run tests based on the results of my x-ray?"

"Yes. You know, it's not normal for a teenage girl not to be able to lay down flat on her back."

"Right..."

"Well, see, you have this mass suppressing you're airway making it difficult for you to breathe. This mass is something we call Hodgkin's Lymphoma Cancer."

My heart stopped, sank, and hesitated on what to do next. My eyes reacted before anything else, releasing a burning sensation of tear drops down my pale, numb, cheeks. My parents instantly walked across the room to hold me, cradle me, cry with me, and assure me that everything was going to be just fine. My immediate response was, "Is it curable?" And her immediate response was, "Highly, highly, curable." An instant, over-whelming, sense of relief washed over my poor, helpless, body. My final words for that moment were, "As long as I'm going to be okay." She assured me I would be in good hands.

The doctor left the room, fully aware that she had just turned our entire world upside down. As my daddy lifted my head up and began to encourage me, giving me examples of people he knew who had fought the same sort of disease and were now perfectly normal, the fear slowly began to melt away. I looked up at my mom and said, "Mom, it's okay. Everything's going to be just fine." One quote that kept replaying itself inside my mind was one by Nick Jonas when he was diagnosed with Type 1 Diabetes, "At first I asked myself 'Why me?', but then I began to ask myself, 'Why not me?'" This really helped me never question why this had to happen to me, because I mean really, why shouldn't this have happened to me? Why should someone else be in my place? I specifically remember directly after all of this in the midst of communicating to my parents that I was okay, making a promise to God. "I'm willing to fight, if you're willing to help. But only if you're willing to help, because I can't do this without you." Ever since that very moment in time, I have plowed forward with faith, confidence, and grace knowing that there is something, or more so someone, bigger and greater than this tumor inside me that is so willing to fight for my life, he gave me his. I'm not exactly sure why God chose me to be the warrior to fight this insane battle, but He did. A lot of people say it's because I'm the bravest person they know. But, you see, it's not me being brave. It's Him showing true bravery through me.

The next couple days were an absolute whirlwind. Saturday and Sunday were probably the two most helpless, hopeless, days of my life. I couldn't sleep, couldn't eat, couldn't think straight. I wasn't grasping reality. They did lots of blood work and had me hooked up to an IV and heart monitor. Monday, Monday, Monday. Ah, Monday was the day of my biopsy. Now, because my lungs were not functioning normally (The example the doctor gave was this: Say your air pipe is supposed to be a size ten, mine was a size two. Your air pipe is supposed to be the size a golf ball and mine was the size of the end of your pinky.), I could not be put under anesthesia. The risk was far too high because it would relax my airways causing them to become more flimsy and not allow air to pass through, ultimately resulting in death. One surgeon (who by the grace of God didn't end up preforming the operation) didn't have a problem saying that to my face either, "I'm just going to be straight forward with you, we can't put you under because you will die." This resulted with an emotional breakdown in my mother's arms directly after.

I had to be awake during the surgery so that I could control my own breathing. The place they were cutting open was my neck. I had to place a lot of trust in the surgeon, being that there are a lot of main blood vessels and such in that location. It was numb, but I was fully there none the less. They offered to give me meds to take the edge off, but I refused because the idea scared me. So, with a sheet over my face and my child life support person beside me to make small talk, the operation began. There was a med student in the room, so the first thing I heard after I was cut open was, "Now, if you look right here you'll see a muscle." Oh. My. Goodness. If that didn't cause me to cringe, I don't know what did. I began to talk and talk with the child life specialist and burn up the un-expected hour and a half I was open. The procedure took longer than expected because he had to go deeper that he thought. Later on, I was thankful because he had extra tissue to donate to research. After the operation he walked out to speak with my parents informing them that he had never seen a teenager so calm and never operated on someone so brave. I was proud to have conquered one of my biggest fears, surgery (and awake at that), and something I have never done before, gotten stitches. But if I were to take the credit for my performance on that operating table, I would be taking something that's not rightfully mine.

Tuesday. I finally thought I could get a day of rest. But, no, instead I have a bone marrow. Bone marrow is the middle part of your bone where all the nerves are located. They had to go in with a needle and pull some out for testing. I was previously warned by some that this process is extremely painful and by others that it hurts terribly but is bearable. Most people my age don't know because they aren't actually awake. They allowed my dad and iPod to come in with me on this one, which made things better. When the first needle went in, I asked my dad if that was it. The iPod was in my ear so I couldn't make out what he was saying but I knew it wasn't a 'yes.' Later on, I found out that first needle was just to numb the skin in that area. I didn't really feel the second needle, which was the first one to go through my hip bone. The third one, however, I felt a lot. The doctor ended up going all the way through my bone and not extracting anything, so he had to pull out and go in again. When all this was going on I didn't know why it hurt so bad, they didn't tell me until I was back in my room. After all of this was done, the anesthesiologist said my "heart rate didn't go past 70". It didn't move up one number, even when the needle went in. He said he was "getting out of here" because he "wasn't needed".

    The few days after this process were more painful than the actual process. The doctor said it would feel like I went ice-skating and fell on my rear. I've been ice-skating, but I've never fallen. So, I described the feeling with a scenario I could actually relate too, "It feels like I went to slide on the softball field but the ground hadn't been rained on for three weeks and I accidentally fell and landed on my hip the wrong way." Days after this whenever I would get a new nurse they would always come in and say "Everyone's talking about you!" or "I heard you are one amazingly tough girl!" I guess they didn't know my biggest fear was needles and things going inside my body that I couldn't control. Like a few months ago, this past summer, when I had my first tic and I cried. I was being held together, but not by my own strength.

Wednesday. As far as I can remember this day was pretty chill. I was pretty nervous all day because we were getting all the results back to see what stage I was and what form of treatment I would need and for how long. When the doctor first came in the room, he said that he looked at the x-ray and the cancer was not in my bones. That was an extreme relief. He then continued to say that it most likely was not in my bone marrow because it wasn't in the blood that came out with the marrow and typically if it's not in one; it's not in the other. This was extremely exciting news because had it been in my bone marrow, I would have automatically jumped to a stage 4 and my survival rate would have dropped to 70%. He had also previously informed us by looking at the CT scan that it had not spread any lower than my chest. Had it gone into my abdomen, I would have been at a stage 3. So, later on that day I was officially diagnosed as a stage 2. They started my first chemo later than expected; it went until about 10:30 at night. They had to slow it down because usually chemo is injected into the body through a stint in your chest, however, they couldn't give me one because of the location of the tumor. So, they had to put it in through my IV. Which was fine for the first three meds, but the fourth med enters the body at an extremely fast pace, and because it was entering through an unusually small vain in my arm as oppose to a larger vain in my chest, the rapid flow was very painful. They ended up having to turn off the chemo and consult a doctor to make sure slowing down the pace wouldn't affect the treatment process. It turns out slowing it down a little was ok but too much does altar the effectiveness of the drug. They put it at a comfortable rate which made the hour and a half process closer to two or two and a half. Another reason it went so late into the evening, I actually ate during chemo. I had a sandwich and a bag of chips. It was rather funny.

My side effects were extremely mild compared to most. I won't go into detail but I can say I never threw up and the other very few side effects were gone within 24 hours. Thursday I just felt exhausted and achy everywhere, and that evening was like PMS on steroids. But besides that, I can't complain. Friday was all about recovery and trying to catch up on lack of sleep. Saturday we had the slim hope of possibly going home, so they took a CT scan to see if my airway had opened up enough. It hadn't. There was great improvement, but they weren't comfortable letting me go home. And because the tumor had started dying it was turning into fluid and the fluid was building up between the left side of my chest and the wall of my left lung. This process is completely normal, but they needed to monitor the fluid to make sure it didn't cause problems. If it became an issue, they would have to stick a needle in between two of my ribs and remove the fluid. I asked the doctor how the fluid is supposed to exit my body on its own, and he said it's just like having a bruise, your body will absorb it on its own (and if it doesn't, in comes the needle.). So, we have to stay put until mid-week. One huge reason being that Cat scans are a lot of radiation on your body, which is bad for anyone but especially females because it nearly doubles your chance of breast cancer long term. Because of this, the doctor wants to use radiation as little as possible especially because I may end up needing that form of treatment towards the end. (It has been one of our biggest prayers that I won't.)

I'm supposed to go home tomorrow. I hope and pray with nearly everything I am that I can go home tomorrow. I have been in this room for twelve straight days now. I've been up and walked around, been to the game room and 'fake' Starbucks, the cafeteria and the gift shop. But none of those places are home.

One amazing thing that happened to me at some point this week was when my mom sat down to read the Bible with me before bed and she randomly opened up to Psalms 91. This scripture has been my rock ever since. I sent out a text message to all of my close family and friends telling them to read it ASAP. The next day a dear friend was at the library in our community college and got a spare moment to open up her Bible and read it. She began to cry.

Psalm 91

"Those who go to God most high for safety will be protected by the Almighty. I will say to the Lord, "You are my place of safety and protection. You are my God and I trust you." God will save you from hidden traps and from deadly diseases. He will cover you with his feathers, and under his wings you can hide. His truth will be your shield and protection. You will not fear any danger by night or an arrow during the day. You will not be afraid of diseases that come in the dark or sickness that strikes at noon. At your side one thousand people may die, or even ten thousand right beside you, but you will not be hurt. You will only watch and see the wicked punished. The Lord is your protection; you have made God most high your place of safety. Nothing bad will happen to you; no disaster will come to your home. He has put his angels in charge of you to watch over you wherever you go. They will catch you in their hands so that you will not hit your foot on a rock.

You will walk on lions and cobras; you will step on strong lions and snakes. The Lord says, 'Whoever loves me, I will save. I will protect those who know me. They will call to me, and I will answer them. I will be with them in trouble; I will rescue them and honor them. I will give them a long, full life, and they will see how I can save.'"

I have already learned so incredibly much from this. More than I ever thought possible. More about me, more about God, more about life, more about my friends and my family, more about the common bond between all Christians, more about cancer, more about why everyone needs to know more. I have learned that you are stronger than you think and braver than you know. That sometimes we're faced with trials in order to build up an unknown sense of courage or discover parts of ourselves we never knew existed. I will never place my change back into my wallet instead of into the CHKD donations box at the Dairy Queen inside of the mall, or anywhere. I will take in every smell, every sight, every sound, every moment. When my fingers slide across the piano, when my mom makes dinner, when my little brother laughs. Things I was deprived of for nearly two weeks. I won't ever hate school work or going to school, I'll just be thankful my body is healthy enough to do the work or go. I will never complain over having a bad hair day, because I may wake up tomorrow and barely have hair. I will never complain because I have an annoying cold, because now I barely have an immune system. I experienced a loss of control over my life, and learned that we all truly have hardly any control at all. Every breath will be used to produce something positive. I learned that I have cancer, and there are still people in this world worse off than I am.

Lastly, I want to thank every single person who sent or left a card, a gift, balloons, a text message, a phone call, a Facebook comment/message, or came to visit. If you did anything to reach out to me or my family, thank you, thank you, thank you. You may not know it, but it means a lot. And for those of you who didn't stop by to see me, thank you as well for giving me and my family time to heal and recover. We are still in that process because as the bad cells are being attacked and destroyed, so are the good cells. Therefore, I don't really have an immune system to fight away illness. I'll still be able to live somewhat like a normal 16 year old; I just have to be a lot more cautious and probably not out in public as much. My treatment plan is laid out for 2 months (for now), going to the clinic every Tuesday but only receiving chemo therapy every other Tuesday. If the tumor is gone, which is our prayer, I'll be done. But I'll have ongoing checkups until I'm 25. If it's not gone, I'll do another round of the same chemo or be treated with radiation therapy. They don't like using radiation therapy on females because it doubles your risk of breast cancer. I'm so ready to get going with this process and have it over and done with. I'm thankful for the things I've gained, but ready to be done because of what I've lost. I suppose my mom's friend said it the best when she described her son's cancer, cancer is a "terrible blessing".

"The Lord is close to the brokenhearted and saves those who are crushed in spirit." Psalms 34:18

There are many memories that stick out to me from being in the hospital. Although I didn't write about all of them in detail while they were occurring, I can still relive them vividly in my mind. These are a few of the experiences I dealt with during my stay in the hospital from the perspective of being in that moment.

Today dad brought some of my stuff from home to me in the hospital. Standing on the cold hard floor in a bathroom so white it almost makes you feel a nonexistent chill, I stared at myself in the mirror. Staring back at me was a face showing how sick I appeared to the rest of the world. Slowly, I put the mascara on adding color to my washed out face. Cancer and color typically don't go hand in hand. I was painted pale with sickness until I made my eyelashes darker. (Or, at least that's the distorted view I had taken and held on to for quite some time. It took a good two solid years for me to be able to look into a mirror wearing no makeup and not see myself standing in a hospital bathroom. Whenever I was without mascara, it reminded me of being sick. I had to retrain my brain.) I put on the mascara, and gained a little bit of confidence. I don't think I ever fully realized at any point what the rest of the world saw when they looked at me.

I haven't taken a shower since my surgery because I'm paranoid to get the bandage or stitches wet. I haven't even removed the bandage to look at the scar. Today mom had to help me wash my hair in the bath so that I wouldn't get the bandage wet. Do you know how humbling it is to be sixteen and have your mom give you bath? At first I was embarrassed but I honestly wasn't up for trying anything on my own. Between the location of the incision being right on my neck and being hooked up to an IV, I was debilitated when it came to washing my own hair.

I finally removed the bandage to look at the scar today. It's pretty small and not extremely noticeable. I kind of just kept staring at it because it's so crazy to think about why it's there. How they opened me up to take cancer out for testing and research, and how I was awake the whole time they did it. I'm trying to take everything in but I feel like I'm in a daze.

Today I didn't think I was going to have to have any tests or anything done, which was fantastic since I've been going non-stop since I got here. However, I was then informed otherwise. First of all, I did not want to go downstairs or to any floor for that matter. Secondly, I most certainly did not need them to wheelchair me down. I'm not sure why, but they didn't give me the option to walk or not. I can't stand that. I'm perfectly capable of walking myself. Then, when I went down there, they hooked all of these wire things to me so they could monitor my heart rate. After that long process, the tech did an ultrasound on my heart. At this point I'm pretty use to having to move my shirt around in uncomfortable ways that most people would find awkward. The gel was cold and she pressed the ultrasound camera extremely hard against me. It wasn't the most pleasant of days and I wasn't in the greatest of moods, unfortunately.

Every night that we've been here my mom's rubbed my back until I fell asleep. Last night I was so miserable and uncomfortable and my mom was so worn out and drained I pushed the button to call in a nurse and literally asked if there was anyone available to rub my back. I didn't mean it in a spoiled rotten kind of way at all, but physical touch is comforting and healing and it's really done so much for me while being here. My child life specialist played with my hair during my bone marrow and my surgery because that is one of the most calming, relaxing, things for me. Another night earlier this week they actually had to put me on oxygen because apparently I was in deep sleep and not breathing well on my own. That was kind of scary because I never would've realized that I was suffocating on my own, and having tubes in your nose isn't really comfortable. The extra oxygen was nice though.

Isn't it funny how people can become memories and lessons to be learned in and of themselves? In the room right beside me is a girl just my age, sixteen. I haven't ever talked to her, but mom and dad do kind of frequently. Then again I guess if I actually left the room a little bit that might increase my odds of socialization. This girl is from Maryland, about three hours away from the hospital. Because of the commute, her parents can't stay with her all of the time, only on weekends. She's fighting leukemia. She has to be in the hospital for three weeks at a time every two weeks for three years. Can you imagine your high school years being spent in a hospital? Not only that, but during the week your parents are at home taking care of your siblings and working to make ends meet as the hospital bills pile up. You only get to see your family on weekends. One day dad was heading out to get me a smoothie from a specific smoothie shop. Before he left, he asked the girl if he could get her anything. She not only said yes, but explained the reason why she wasn't quite sure what she wanted. Right before she was admitted to the hospital, her daddy was supposed to take her there. She had still never been. Every part of this girl's situation breaks my heart. Not only that, but it keeps me thankful. Even though I'm in the hospital fighting cancer, I know it won't be for as long as this young lady has to take residence here. I have my parent's 24/7 and I'm only twenty minutes away from home. Her parents can only see her on weekends and she's three hours away from everything she knows. This young lady is one of my first examples in seeing that there's always someone who's fighting a battle more or equally complicated as your own.

The doctor came in and told me that I need to get up and walk around some today. The thing is, I really have no motivation. I'm quite comfortable lying in this bed staring at these same walls. I mean, there's nothing to go see, I don't really want people seeing me like this, it's irritating and uncomfortable to lug around an IV especially when it beeps like crazy when you're running low on fluid. I can't process anything that's happening because it's all coming so fast. I guess I'm so drained I feel like just laying here is the most logical thing to do. I can't think outside of this room. What's going on at home? What are my siblings doing right now? What are other people thinking? How much do they know? Are they afraid?

As soon as I came home from the hospital, I already had something weighing heavily on my heart. Despite walking into my room and being greeted by a beautiful, homemade, "Welcome Home Lexi" banner, skillfully put together by my sister and our friend LeahAnn, I was still a little distraught. One of the first challenging things I had to do was prepare myself to break the news of my diagnosis over the phone to one of my dearest friends, Allison. Allison and I met at our homeschool group when I was a Freshman in high-school and we're still very close. As difficult and confusing as that circumstance was, I needed her to know and we weren't going to see each other in person any time soon. I remember standing in my room thinking of ways I could bring it up or what I could say to make it seem like the situation wasn't as crippling as it seemed. Eventually I realized that you can't really dull down a life threatening diagnosis. Once I scrounged up enough courage to make the phone call, I didn't beat around the bush. She was astounded, just like everyone else had been.

Besides the lovely banner, another obvious thing I noticed was how immaculately clean our house was. During my hospital stay, my dad had scrubbed and disinfected every square inch of anything I might potentially come in contact with. I remember sitting at dinner the first night I was home; it was so bizarre. After the emotional blessing before we ate, my dad began explaining things to my siblings like, "You have to wash your hands extremely well before you stick them in a bag of chips or anything like that. Alexis can't eat after anyone because of the spread of germs." Realistically speaking, no one in my family ended up washing their hands every time they ate potato chips. The whole "spreading of germs" thing really affected me throughout the whole process. I felt very alienated, actually. Our family dog passed away not long after I finished treatment, and even then when I went to be near her as she was dying, my dad was hesitant. This upset me not only because our beloved dog was passing, but also because I could still feel the disease affecting my life in some ways. I didn't like the idea of cancer or cancer treatment affecting me or how I live my life other than how I chose to apply the experience. Once again I was experiencing a loss of control, and that bothered me.

One of the first specific rules my parent's set was no hugging. Now, for most people that might not be much of an issue, but I am a very affectionate person and it was by no means an easy task for me. The first time I went back to the gym where we played basketball, one of my friends saw me, yelled my name from across the room, ran up to me, and gave me a huge hug. Naturally, I hugged back. A friend that was standing beside me yelled, "GERMS!" which left everyone around (especially the people who had no idea I had just gotten out of the hospital due to cancer) a little confused. She explained to the person hugging me that I was not a loud to hug anyone because of the germ risk. From that day forward, my friends and I coined the term "germs", and would frequently use it as a joke randomly yelling, "GERMS!".

Later on during treatment, I actually started taking shots every day to boost my immune system. Every week when they would draw blood and check my white blood cell count, it would be through the roof. I went from one extreme to the other, from not being able to touch people to being "invincible", eventually being called "Superwoman".

The other day my mom, Miss Amy, and I were talking about how much I've changed because of all of this and the difference between a child going thru it and a teenager. (Because Miss Amy's son, Zach, had cancer at the young age of two but I was sixteen.) I said that one of the biggest things for me was that as a teenager I naturally felt invincible, I felt like nothing could hurt me. Then all of a sudden, BAM! You're fighting for your life. It made me realize I had absolutely no control. I was at an utter and total loss of power. Miss Amy then asked a really good question, "Well, now that you're beating it do you feel more powerful or less?"

That was a tricky question for me, but I responded with...

"In some ways I feel stronger, like now after this I feel like I can do anything. But in other ways, I feel completely out of control. Like I can never really control what is going to happen, only how I respond."

Sometimes, you feel different, separate, distant, far away, fake, alone, like you barely exist, so invisible you could be swept away by the wind. It can fill up your mind like water fills a bath tub. Drowning your thoughts and draining your emotions, causing your heart to sink to your feet. You feel overwhelmed and confused. It doesn't make sense. You can't even say the words because you feel like a liar.

You've never felt this way before

I don't understand

It can consume you.

Deep, deep, within to the most silent, unused, shadowed, places of your inner-being, you begin to discover a place you never knew existed, a strength you didn't know was possible, and a bravery you've never felt before take over. Slowly you begin to unravel the mystery of your much needed inner superhero.

Cancer not only pushed everything into perspective, it was conformation of what was really important in my life. I have to have it. I play it, I sing it, I teach it, I breathe it. I confirmed that sharing the passion of music is what I want to do for a living by teaching, and that music really can help heal a broken heart.

(After leading kids worship, I have decided to combine some of my greatest passions: children, ministry, and worship through music. I'm headed more in the direction of music ministry as oppose to teaching piano now, even though I'm still doing both.)

    I have learned the meaning of true friendship and spending the night in instead of going out. It started when I was stuck in the hospital and was craving white pizza, so my wonderful Aunt JoAnne brought me some and joined my mom and I for dinner. That was a true girl's night in.

THE ART OF GIRLS' NIGHT

At some moment in time, in some place in this world, some person in history said, "Life isn't about waiting for the storm to pass; it's about learning to dance in the rain." I have found this to be extremely true and relevant no matter what storm you're caught in. Every day is about making the best things in life happen, not the worst things getting in the way.

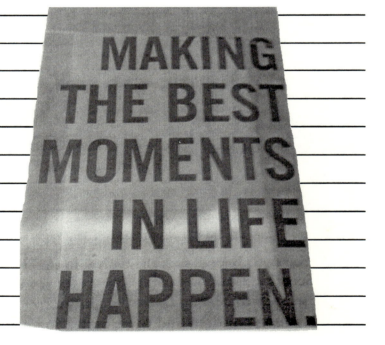

MAKING THE BEST MOMENTS IN LIFE HAPPEN.

"Why, you do not even know what will happen tomorrow. What is your life? You are a mist that appears for a little while and then vanishes." James 4:14

February 11th, 2010

    My body is in a war against itself. That doesn't scare me, but it hurts sometimes. There are moments when I break down and feel so weak and helpless and I think to myself, "If they could see me now, would they feel the same way?" Would people still think that I'm one of the strongest people they know if they saw the tears streaming down my cheeks and soaking my pillow or making a path down my hands? Then I have to remind myself that **strength is not an emotion that eliminates fear, but rather an emotion that helps you overcome your fear.** True strength is crying until you have no more tears, admitting to yourself that you are petrified of something, facing what scares you the most no matter how small and insecure it makes you feel, and ultimately rising above your fear. Not to say that you have no fear, but rather saying that you now have the courage to battle the fear. I have chemo to battle my cancer, but what about my heart and mind? What do I have to battle with that? Strength, courage, faith, hope, and love. I have strength deep inside me I never knew existed. I have a type of courage you could only gain when you've seen death face-to-face. I have faith that can overcome anything I'll ever go through in life again. I have a hope that everything is going to be absolutely fine. And, I have love, because in the words of Jesus himself, "...the greatest of these is love." The greatest thing you could ever give another person is love. The greatest thing that has brought me through all of this is love. The only reason I don't feel like a complete and total failure when I'm crying until my tears melt the world away, is because of His love.

"But God demonstrates his own love for us in this: While we were still sinners, Christ died for us."

Romans 5:8

I have been taught the power of prayer. I have been reminded that when you talk to God he really is listening, and sometimes it's nice to know there really is someone who completely understands. I have lived through a difficult season and never ceased to rejoice. I have proven that when God says to praise him in the times of trouble, it's because He wants to bless you for it.

PRAY

REJOICE!

When you're getting chemo, they have to flush you're line (the tube connected to the IV giving you the medicine) with saline to make sure it's not only clean but working the way it should. Eventually, you become nauseated from the taste of the saline. For me personally it was not as strong of a taste going into my arm as it was the port in my chest, probably because your chest is much closer to your mouth. (A port is a piece of rubber placed in a main vein typically either in your chest or on your side used to access the vein easily and pump the chemo into your body and draw blood for blood work. Because these veins are larger than the ones in your arms, the process is not only faster but also much less painful.) I remember my nurse coming over and actually saying something about the fact that I hadn't gotten sick from it yet, because that was highly unusual. I think she might've even been anticipating it being that she had the bucket ready. Anyways, I'm not even sure she finished voicing her thought and I was already vomiting. What's odd is the average person can't "taste" saline whenever they have blood drawn or an IV put in. I only began to taste it over a period of time, like most cancer patients. What's fantastic is on the second floor where the clinic is located, once you can taste the saline and you discover you can't stomach it any longer, they flush with sugar water instead. To this day I chew gum before scans to disguise the taste as much as possible because for some reason on the first floor (where they do CT scans) they only use saline.

Speaking of ports, that might've been one of the longest, toughest fights I've ever put up. Up until that point, I hadn't been knocked out for any form of surgery and I wasn't planning on it. I was absolutely avoiding it at all costs. Eventually though, the cost was painstakingly high for everyone around me. The veins in my arms began to basically shut down as far as being available for IV access. They would not only roll (causing me to be stuck by needles countless times in one sitting), but once they got the needle into the vein, more times than not they wouldn't be able to draw blood. If by some chance they were able to draw blood and get the IV going, it wasn't long until my hand and/or arm was experiencing immense pain.

I can remember the hand hooked up to the IV was always ice cold and I would put heat packs on it. (As I often did before getting stuck with a needle in order to get my blood flowing. I had a whole routine, like drinking plenty of liquids and making fists with my hands.) It was also very painful because there are many tiny veins in your hands and the drugs were entering my body at a very rapid pace. Often times I could feel the medicine going up my forearm. Just thinking about that feeling makes me nauseated to this day. It would take all afternoon for me to finish getting the treatment when it was only supposed to take a few hours.

Eventually, my mom, the nurses, and the child life specialists, (but mostly my mom) couldn't handle seeing me in that much pain anymore. I remember the day the child life specialist came into the room to talk to me about getting a port. My doctor had told me that as long as it was okay with the nurses I didn't have to get a port, but if they started having problems I'd have to get one put in. I really didn't have much of a choice at this point. There was no other way for me to receive treatment and my veins were failing me. I was receiving treatment while having this conversation, and I was completely miserable. My mom was outside of the room on the phone with my dad and he actually came in to see me. (That was the only time my dad came to the hospital after I was initially released, simply because there was never a need for him and it was healthier to have a small amount of people in the clinic where kids received chemo. It decreases the risk of germ spread. My dad showing up immediately indicated my mom's desperate need to have him there to help convince me.)

Against everything I wanted, I ended up having the surgery to have the port put in. Shockingly, I was immediately grateful. I received chemo directly after the surgery and the entire chemotherapy process was so much smoother, faster, and pain free. I didn't have to be poked at a million times or feel the fluid rush through my veins. In a way, I wish I had gotten the port sooner. (Directly after this surgery before receiving treatment, I was offered the opportunity to meet a few professional hockey players that were visiting the hospital. Being a sixteen year old girl coming off of anesthesia, I said no. I wasn't up for it, didn't feel well, and even though I wasn't processing completely normally I knew I didn't look well. Mostly because I knew what was coming with the treatment.)

Surgery

I've talked to a lot of people about their experience being put to sleep before a surgery, and hardly any of them remember as much as I do. I remember having thoughts running through my head like, "What if I don't wake up?" Or, my biggest fear, "What if I'm awake while its going on but I'm so numb I can't tell them?" Watching shows on TV isn't a good idea when they're based off of real events that involve things like those thoughts. My mom told me not to worry, because it will be the best sleep I've ever had. And it was. Right before I went out, I remember everything...

I remember picking my flavor laughing gas, watermelon. I remember the bright lights. I remember the lady and what she said, "Okay, Alexis, I want you to slowly breathe and just relax. Now this is gonna kinda make your fingers and toes tickle a little, and when it does, I want you to tell me." I instantly moaned, to numb to even utter words. She then replied with, "Wow! Already? You're a cheap date! Now I'm gonna turn it up a little and I want you to breathe in as deep as you can and then slowly exhale like you're blowing out a candle." As I started to do what she asked, the blinding lights started to blur like they do on all the movies and TV shows. Then, I started to think about how it was working and I was going down. I told myself, "Dang, Alexis, you're not even gonna get to finish blowing out the candle." Almost at the same time she assured me that I was doing great and before I knew it I'd be waking up and it would all be over with. Then, I said to myself, "Okay, Alexis, here it is. You're going out." And that was it.

The day before my port surgery, the Brock family gave me a ring. I wanted it to be the last thing I looked at before I was knocked out, but you aren't allowed to wear jewelry in the O.R. I kept the plastic the ring came on which is pictured below. The actual ring says "Love life Be brave". I found it outstandingly symbolic of everything I have been through and stand for.

Love the life you have been given, and be thankful you have been given life. Be courageous no matter what your life throws at you, even if you don't think you can handle it. Follow your dreams, make them a reality. Don't let your circumstances define who you are or what you become. Allow them to shape you into the best person you can be.

Love life

Love Life
Be Brave

Whenever you wear this ring
remember; be courageous, follow
your dreams and love life.

LONG LIVE *Life*

Tuesday, March 23rd, 2010

It's been a while since I've written anything. I'm so bad with this kind of stuff, journaling and such. I'm supposed to be keeping a frequent journal but I'm just so busy. I guess that's not a bad thing though, because it obviously means things are good enough to where I can have a normal life. This is going to be another long one. I guess I just like making a few really long ones as opposed to a bunch of really short ones.

I got treatment today. As I was sitting on the bed thinking about how gross it was that they had just stuck a needle in my chest to access my port, this little boy went by with a nurse and a child life specialist. He was coming from the back where the toys and PlayStations are and such and they were bribing him to go up front superfast so they could either draw blood or access his port. As they walked past where I was sitting the small child began to let out a long, drawn out, moan full of fear and uncertainty. Seconds later it turned into short breaths and tiny, little, helpless, whimpers. It sounded exactly the way my little brothers sound when they are about to be significantly punished. But then I realized this child has done absolutely nothing wrong. Not to say he's perfect, but to say he has done nothing to deserve this life threating illness and life draining treatment process. No human being deserves that. Every single Tuesday I witness the sight of young children fighting for their lives with smiles on their faces, and those kids are my heroes.

A few weeks ago I was reading in the paper about how they found the killer to that innocent teenage girl who was murdered in her kitchen about a year ago in Portsmouth. The paper had listed everything the police had to investigate to solve the crime. The amount of research was ridiculous. But then when I read out the list to my dad I ended by saying, "That seems like so much, but I bet to everyone who knew her, it was never enough." He added on by saying "or fast enough." Then I thought about cancer research, and about how to me and those who loved me it was an important cause, but now, it's not important enough. It's my life saver. Thoughts started taking over my open mind filling it to the brim with hurt for those in which cancer research wasn't fast or accurate enough. For that teenage girl, the research was done so she would not die in vain. For me, the research is done so I will not live in vain.

I began talking with my dad and we were discussing how much violence is in this evil world and it's gotten to the point to where we hardly care. I mean think back 50 or 60 years, a stolen car would have sent the whole part of town into a frantic mode. Now, we have such bigger problems with our society we've just accepted the fact that cars will get stolen. But you see the thing about all this is, it doesn't really and truly begin affecting you until it's brought into your living room. In your mind; People stealing cars is just something that happens this day in age. Until it's your car that's missing from your driveway. Maybe that teenager should have made a better choice in friends or had more parental supervision. Until that teenager is one that use to dwell in or visit your living room. Vandalism is just what punks will do. There's no way to stop them really. It's too out of control. Until it's your garage they spray paint. Cancer is so curable with all the meds they have now. Until the person you love is told they're fighting for their life. It's so unlikely for a child to get cancer, I mean really I don't think it happens that much. Maybe I should save my change for another research foundation or for my own family, I mean times are tough. Until it's your child that needs the change for the research to save their life. See, my dad and I, we realized that through this whole process, we've had a revelation. Something won't bother you half as much if it's not brought into your living room.

So now, I have a new heart and compassion for others. Not that I wasn't loving before or anything, but my entire perspective on good and evil has changed. Bad things happen to good people, that's just a part of life. You take the bad with the good and celebrate what you do have instead of what you're "missing". I've learned that as my Pastor says it, "The measure of her response was the measure of her blessing." Depending on how you respond to all life throws at you is how you can determine the outcome. And just because something doesn't affect you or someone you love in a personal way, it doesn't mean that the exact same thing isn't causing someone else's whole world to fall apart.

P.S.

Happy birthday to the most incredible woman in the world; my mother. I'm so happy I could eat lunch with you and didn't get sick from treatment until after (like when I was writing this). This has to be harder on you than on me, I just cannot imagine watching your own child go thru so much. You never once fail to amaze me. When I grow up, I wanna be just like you!

I love you mommy.

"Many women do noble things, but you surpass them all."

Proverbs 31:29

49

Mom and I on Easter Sunday, 2010

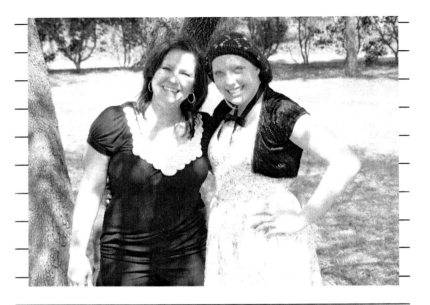

Mom and I on Easter Sunday, 2011

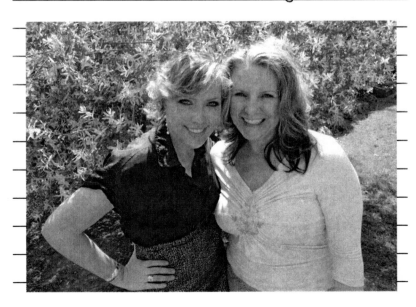

Tuesday, March 30th, 2010

On Tuesday, March 30th, 2010, I had a clinic visit. This was the day we were going to get the Doctor's "Okay" to go on our vacation to Florida in May from the 8th-15th. We had planned a year in advance and had extended family going with us. I just remember sitting in the clinic praying to myself, "Dear Jesus, please help me to be able to go to Disney world, please. Amen." Over and over again. We ended up getting the "Okay". But had it been any other date, we wouldn't have been able to go. I also found out that I would be receiving radiation from the time we got back until the middle of June. Five days a week for a month. The one and only month this summer that isn't slam packed. God really knows how to deal with details.

Thoughts

A lot of people have told me that I don't belong here and I don't deserve this. However, I would have to disagree. To me, that's like telling a solider that he doesn't belong in a war. If a solider doesn't belong in a war, then where does he belong? This is my battle, and telling me I don't belong in it defeats the purpose of what I was made for. Soldiers were made to fight their battles and I was made to fight mine. If I wasn't made for this, I wouldn't be doing it or defeating it. You can't win every battle and sometimes you lose a soldier, but that doesn't mean they weren't exactly where they were supposed to be doing everything they should have been to the best of their potential.

There was a time in my life when I was utterly afraid to fall asleep. Afraid that once I closed my eyes I would never wake to see the light of day again. Afraid that whatever thought was the last to capture my attention before I drifted away into unconsciousness would be the very last thing my mortal mind comprehended. I was afraid of being the judge of my own wellbeing. The doctors were gone, the nurses weren't checking my vital signs every hour, there was no band around my finger connected to a machine to make sure my heart was beating regularly, there was no IV to make sure I had enough fluid to sustain life. I was on my own. I'm the only one who can tell how I feel, but I didn't even think I was sick in the first place, let alone dying. What if I started dying again? Who would save me then? What if this time we weren't so lucky and it was too late? But then I realized something. We're all dying. Every day we get even closer. Why should I spend my nights lying in bed wondering if I'll ever wake up again? I should spend my nights in confidence knowing that I'm going to be okay. I should dream about the future I long for, knowing that I possess the power to turn it into a reality. So that's what I did.

"I have told you these things, so that in me you might have peace. In this world you will have trouble. But take heart! I have overcome the world."

John 16:33

Right now I'm thinking about the moment I was diagnosed, when the doctor told me what I had. I could only hold on to her last three words, "Hodgkin's Lymphoma Cancer." It was as if my brain automatically separated the words into two parts, "Hodgkin's Lymphoma" and "cancer". I tried to focus on the side of my brain that was clutching to "Hodgkin's Lymphoma", because my lack of knowledge in the oncology area made it impossible for me to relate that term to cancer. The word I was avoiding to prevent being petrified. I think everyone when forced with a problem has this little piece of themselves that just wants to forget everything and run to the far ends of the earth. My automatic response was to first tell the doctor "No.", that she was wrong. The test results and x-rays belonged to someone else in the hospital. But not me. I wasn't the one with cancer. And secondly, after being told I was the one who was wrong, then I would run. But within the time span of a minute, a minute that felt like centuries had passed, I realized that this was reality and it was happening right here and right now and I couldn't run away. Running away from your problems doesn't make them go away. If I did run away, my cancer would still be inside me taking my life by the second.

"When I called, you answered me; you greatly emboldened me."

Psalm 138:3

Anyone who is close to me knows that I cannot tolerate a complaining spirit. My mom always taught my siblings and I that anyone can find the negative in a situation, that's not hard. But it takes someone special to find the positive. People complain about things that are so inferior to other issues in the world and I absolutely do not understand how. I think it has to do with where we're at as a society. We are consumers. We want what we want, when we want it, how we want it. We're so use to having things right at the tips of our fingers. Sometimes, we must die to self. Look at the big picture; two weeks from now, ten months from now, twenty-five years from now, will your circumstances matter? It's not what's going on around you that will live on when people think about you; it's what you did about it. How you react to negativity says everything about you. In the heat of the fire a person's true colors are displayed. It shows a lost and dying world that even in the midst of chaos there is peace. When you're confronted with a negative situation and things don't go your way, how do you handle it differently than someone who doesn't know Christ? You're a testimony at all times. Does your testimony point people towards the hope of Jesus?

"Be devoted to one another in love. Honor one another above yourselves."

Romans 12:10

"Be joyful always; pray continually; give thanks in all circumstances, for this is God's will for you in Christ Jesus."

1 Thessalonians 5:16-18

"The human spirit can endure in sickness, but a crushed spirit who can bear?"

Proverbs 18:14

"A cheerful heart is good medicine, but a crushed spirit dries up the bones."

Proverbs 17:22

Some people don't understand how everything was back to normal after I was told my disease was highly curable and I was going to be okay. I think they can't comprehend it because literally just moments before I had been diagnosed. So, I'll try and explain this as well as I can. When you're told out of nowhere, totally unexpectedly, that you have something inside your body that is taking away your life every minute and you have absolutely no control over it yourself, everything around you disappears and in your mind you watch as your whole world suddenly bursts into shatters. You only have one priority, getting the killer out. But, when you're told just a few moments later, after you've been to the lowest point known to mankind, looking death in the face, that you're gonna be okay after your first priority is accomplished; that's when nothing else truly matters. Because within five minutes I felt what it was like to have your life taken away and given back again. Those five minutes changed my perspective on my entire life.

I don't like to think under the terms of 'One person can only do so much.' I like to think under the terms of 'Only one person can do so much.'

"Now to him who is able to immeasurably more than all we ask or imagine, according to his power that is at work within us..."

Ephesians 3:20

Those five minutes changed my life because they completely changed the way I view life. Every situation is now looked at from a perspective that the majority of people aren't capable of comprehending until the end of their life. When most people replay their life and have flashbacks of certain events and people that meant the most to them, it's after they've lived a long, full, life. That just wasn't the case for me. I was sixteen when I thought my life was coming to an end. In that moment when I was told I had cancer, in my mind's eye everything in my life literally just disappeared. The only thing left was people. That moment completely changed everything because it showed me that when I'm at the end of my life and I look back, whatever car I drove, whatever shirt someone spilt something on and ruined, whatever TV episodes my DVR did or didn't record, whatever softball game I won or lost, those things don't matter at all. These are the things that make or break our positive attitudes on a day-to-day basis. Frustration over lost keys, traffic, or the trash not being taken out; those things mean absolutely nothing. I'm not saying we should live irresponsible lives with no drive or organization. I'm not saying that at all. In fact, a short life is all the more reason to live accordingly. All I'm saying is that when you're at the end of your life the things that are going to either be breaking your heart or making you feel like you actually accomplished something with the time you had, it all comes down to the way you treated people. Most importantly the ones you love the most, because those are the people that were left in my mind when I thought I was going to die. I thought to myself, "If I died right now, what would those people think about me? Would they feel loved or would they just remember all the times I became irritated and short-tempered with them? How did I impact their life? Did my words build them up or tear them down? Did I even make a difference? Will it even affect them if I'm gone?" I am so thankful that I had the opportunity to experience what it's like to be at the end of your life without actually being there. I was completely there mentally and emotionally, even if it was only for a matter of minutes. Those minutes totally redefined my relationships, the way I treat people, and the way I live my life. It made me think about how I want to be remembered after I'm gone.

I will NOT PACK MY WORRIES. I WILL NOT PLAN ANYTHING PAST TODAY. I WILL SURPRISE MYSELF.

I WILL BE THE TORTOISE, NOT THE HARE. I WILL ENGAGE IN A THREE-HOUR CONVERSATION ABOUT NOTHING IN PARTICULAR. I WILL ACT FIRST AND THINK LATER. I WILL QUIT BEING MYSELF. I will live life to the fullest.

I will not pack my worries.

I will not remind myself of what I need not worry.

"Therefore do not worry about tomorrow, for tomorrow will worry about itself. Each day has enough trouble of its own."
Matthew 6:34

"Are not two sparrows sold for a penny? Yet not one of them will fall to the ground outside your Father's care. And even the very hairs of your head are all numbered. So don't be afraid; you are worth more than many sparrows."
Matthew 10:29-31

I will not plan past today.

I will live in this moment.

I will be the tortoise, not the hare.

I will soak up every minute of every day and not let life pass me by. I will make every attempt to slow down time and learn from every experience.

"Teach us to number our days, that we may gain a heart of wisdom."

Psalms 90:12

"Wisdom is a shelter as money is a shelter, but the advantage of knowledge is this: Wisdom preserves those who have it."

Ecclesiastes 7:12

I will quit being myself.

I will think of others by putting myself in their shoes and consider what they're going through and be thankful for what I have and who I am.

"Be devoted to one another in love. Honor one another above yourselves."

Romans 12:10

I will live life to the fullest.

I think this one pretty much explains itself.

I will engage in a three hour conversation about nothing in particular.

Life is too short not to spend time just simply talking to the ones you love.

I will act first and think later.

I will take risks without letting fear take control.

Is it possible for someone to ever be prepared to be told they have cancer? I don't really think so. When I think about how sudden I was told, I use to often think, "Would it have been any less painful if I had already been thinking it was a possibility?" But to be honest, I think the sting was a lot shorter because of the shock.

Is it possible for someone to ever be fully prepared to battle cancer? I don't really think so. Even though I have felt fully able since I was told I'd have to. In my mind it just wasn't optional. You can make your problem better or worse but it is what it is.

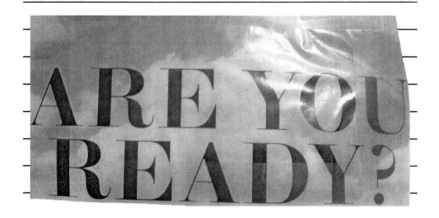

When dealing with a trial, it may be easy for one to think negatively and pursue life hopelessly. However, I see trial as a golden opportunity to discover and allow your view to change. It is like an exercise of the mind and spirit, creating weakness to build strength. Giving opportunity to cleanse yourself of un-needed emotions.

THE VIEW CHANGES

A golden opportunity to discover

"And whatever you do, whether in word or deed, do it all in the name of the Lord Jesus, giving thanks to the Father through Him. Whatever you do, work at it with all your heart, as working for the Lord, not human masters..."

Colossians 3:17, 23

Did you know you're absolutely gorgeous? Did you know your smile and your heart radiate so brightly they make the darkness run and hide? Your inner beauty chases away any lack of confidence you may be covering up. You were designed to portray the maker of the stars. How could you not be stunning? Learning to carry yourself with confidence in knowing who you are and class that separates you from the rest of the world, that's what makes you pretty. (This was written at a time when I was feeling slightly insecure about the amount of hair loss caused by chemotherapy.)

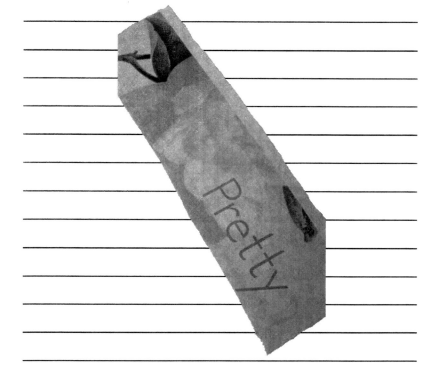

"I also want women to dress modestly, with decency and propriety, adorning themselves, not with elaborate hairstyles or gold or pearls or expensive clothes, but with good deeds, appropriate for women who profess to worship God."

1 Timothy 2:9-10

"For you created my inmost being; you knit me together in my mother's womb. I praise you because I am fearfully and wonderfully made; your works are wonderful, I know that full well."

Psalm 139:13-14

In my mind I can vividly remember a moment when I was sitting on my hospital bed bawling as my mom held me. There were probably many different things that contributed to that break down, but the one thought that's branded in my mind is my first high school prom. I was looking forward to my first opportunity to go to prom that year with a group of girls I was friends with, but I realized that by that time I wouldn't have any hair. As I began to picture myself taking prom pictures bald, I was traumatized.

One of the first nights I stayed in the hospital I felt this unexplainable, supernatural, peace about losing my hair before the process of losing it started. I've never felt anything quite like it before. At the time, I interpreted that peace as meaning I wasn't going to lose any of my hair at all. Earlier that day I had been talking to someone who was encouraging me about potentially losing my hair. The next morning, I actually texted them and asked if God had told them that night I wasn't going to lose it, because I was given a supernatural peace unlike anything I've ever experienced before. They said no, God didn't tell them that, but everything would be okay.

In retrospect, I can see how God was giving me supernatural peace and telling me that everything was going to be okay and I manipulated that promise to my version of "okay". Not intentionally but through misinterpretation. In my eyes, in that moment, the only "okay" option was to not lose my hair. But God knew that everything would in fact be okay if I lost my hair. This lesson blessed me so much because I now realize that I can't trust my vision of "okay". Instead, I have to trust God's.

In Matthew 6:9-13, the Lord's prayer, there's a line that says "Your will be done". We're called to pray that God's will be done instead of our own because God knows what's best for us. God knew that through Him I could handle losing all of my hair at sixteen; even though to me that seemed nothing short of devastating. God knows what we need in every area of our life all the way down to the tiniest of details, and we need to embrace the fact that that need might not be what we think or feel it is. Never confuse the promise of hope with the promise of your dreams coming true. The promise of hope is new life in Christ because of his choice to buy us with his great love. Because he bought us, that means his vision and his will for our lives. Not our own.

"I have been crucified with Christ and **I no longer live**, but **Christ lives in me**. The life I now live in the body, I live by faith in the Son of God, who loved me and gave himself for me."

Galatians 2:20

"'For my thoughts are not your thoughts, neither are your ways my ways,' declares the Lord. 'As the heavens are higher than the earth, so are my ways higher than your ways and my thoughts higher than your thoughts.'"

Isaiah 55:8-9

Looking back at pictures now, you can see where my eyebrows began to thin out. (I never noticed I lost my eyebrows until I was off of treatment and I was looking through pictures.) I can also look back at pictures and tell when my hair started thinning out. I never lost all of my hair, I ended up shaving what little bit I had left by myself in my bedroom because it was just frustrating and I wanted it to all grow back even. A few months before I was diagnosed, I convinced my mom to buy me a hat that was still full price. Neither one of us ever buys anything at full price. That hat was never removed from my head during treatment except when I was sleeping. It didn't come off my head until all of my hair started growing back in. I think it's safe to say it paid for itself.

One day as my mom and I entered the hospital, we had quite an encounter with the lady at the front desk. We were waiting for the elevator as she asked us what floor we were headed to. This question wasn't out of the ordinary by any means. It was simply a mandatory safety precaution. However, that's not all she asked. She began to explain to me how she remembered my "beautiful, long, blonde hair" and then proceeded to ask me if I would take my hat off. Yes, I know. Unbelievable, right? Ask a sixteen year old girl who's fighting cancer, going through chemo therapy, and clearly has no hair to take her hat off. Not to mention you work at a hospital and encounter patients just like me every day! I was floored and speechless. I didn't know what to say or how to react. Instinctively, I ignored her and proceeded onto the elevator. Mom ended up calling the hospital later to inform them of their interrogative front desk worker.

On another occasion involving my hair, I was eating at Cracker Barrel with a group of friends and this particular girl also took it upon herself to make commentary regarding my hair. I was actually wearing a wig and my hat that evening, and even though I can't remember exactly what her remarks were I remember how they impacted me. It was humiliating. Everyone around knew what I was going through and that my hair had been thinning out, and she took it upon herself to point out that my hair was different. Not different as in I had changed it, different as in unnatural. I'm pretty sure at that point everyone realized it was a wig if they hadn't already. Once again I was caught off guard and left speechless.

I remember the first day I took that hat off. Standing in my room staring in the mirror debating whether or not I had enough hair to where people couldn't tell I had just finished chemotherapy. The last thing I wanted to do was draw attention to myself and the last thing any teenager wants is to stick out and feel alone. It was the middle of June, really hot, and my family was swimming in our pool. I eventually decided that I wanted to go swimming. Really swimming. Not standing in the three foot end with my hat still on. I wanted to be free.

That was a huge, huge, step of courage for me. I was extremely self-conscious. I still have the picture I took exposing everyone to my new hair in the summer of 2010. My hair ended up coming in much thicker and curlier than before. At first, I was rocking a fohawk. Whenever people would complement my "hair cut", my mom would always joke around and say "I don't think they realize how expensive it was."

Chemotherapy actually has the potential to change everything about your hair, and I had heard crazy stories. I had even heard one about a person who previously had gray hair but it grew back with no gray. I was thankful that my hair color didn't change. Also, while I was in the hospital a friend told me that it would take about two years for my hair to grow back to the length it was before I started losing it. I found that theory pretty accurate. I've never been more excited to have long hair.

It's time for me to face the crowd one more time. And something about this just doesn't feel right. I try and give all I am, but no matter how hard I try I never feel like I can. I'm not giving up, I'm just giving in. I can't always be brave, I can't always pretend. I've put on this smile for more than a while, now it's getting the best of this child. This makes me someone I'm not. I wanna be happy but now I've forgot. I get so wrapped up in the emotions involved, then I get lost and I'm not me at all.

This paragraph was written at a time when my hormones were being drastically affected by the drugs given through chemo. I became extremely emotional, which wasn't typical for me at all. It made me feel very much unlike myself, which I couldn't stand. That initial moment of complete surrender that I made to God in the E.R. that night telling Him that I didn't mind fighting cancer but only if He was willing to help, that moment repeated itself multiple times throughout my treatment and still affects me today. In fact, with everything in life I believe we have to learn to give it over to God, otherwise we will not be fully at peace or capable of handling it on our own. Looking back, I'm tempted to erase this. But then I realized you can never erase the past or reality or what you once felt. It's what makes you who you are.

I suppose sometimes crying is the bravest thing and in our weakest moments we are truly the strongest.

"But he said to me, 'My grace is sufficient for you, for my power is made perfect in weakness.' Therefore I will boast all the more gladly about my weakness, so that Christ's power may rest on me."
2 Corinthians 12:9

This may be a little graphic for some, but I can remember the first time I really vomited from treatment. The steroids were making me hungry (as always) and I was craving a chocolate chip cookie and coffee. Being that I had never gotten sick from treatment, my mom went down to the first level of the hospital to try and retrieve the things I was craving. She came back with the closest things she could find, a piece of chocolate cake and a cappuccino from the Starbucks in the lobby. Long story short, neither one stayed down for long and I haven't had either one since. I also haven't had Saltine crackers because that was what I snacked on during treatment. It's challenging when you have steroids going into your body making you abnormally hungry, but at the same time you have a medicine that causes everything you eat to come back up. Sometimes, I would be on nausea pills up to two or three days at a time after receiving treatment. Eventually, just going to the hospital would make me nauseous even if I wasn't getting treatment. It was just as much a mental battle as it was physical. Being in that environment, smelling certain things, hearing certain things, it was all related to chemotherapy and how that affected me. I ended up having to take medicine before every visit, regardless of what I was going for. The idea of going to the hospital made me anxious even after I was in remission, simply because of the trauma that was experienced there.

Whenever I would go in for a doctor appointment my doctor would check random things due to the possible side effects from chemo. While I was undergoing treatment and even some time after, I felt like there was a spot on my leg that had no feeling. It doesn't bother me anymore, so I'm assuming whatever was causing it wore off. Totally weird.

Every single time I ever went in to talk to the doctor while going through the course of treatment my mom was with me. Of course, naturally, with any good mother comes an abundance of concern and a lot of questions. For some reason, my mom was always really great at thinking of new questions to ask the doctor, even when I insisted she just keep them to herself (mostly because I was afraid of some of the answers). My doctor always said that other than my mom, there was this one other mom who was just so concerned. Not that it was a bad thing, just funny. One of those embarrassing "parent" moments happened when my dad made a mandatory request that I ask the doctor if I was a loud to use bug spray. According to him, it's extremely potent. I guess he assumed that every person undergoing chemotherapy just didn't go outside because they'd be carried away by mosquitos, I'm not exactly sure. But my doctor and I got a good laugh out of it. (On a side note, I don't really use typical bug spray anymore. It is in fact very potent, and this whole experience has made me even more health cautious than I was before. I honestly think we can attribute the chemicals in bug spray to many diseases today, just like the chemicals in cleaning products, nail polish, etc.

There's this one story that really impacted my dad when I was sick, and I'm pretty sure he still reflects on it frequently. We have an in-ground pool in our backyard and in the flower bed surrounding it we have these huge rocks. One day, during the time frame I was going through chemotherapy, I helped my dad unload the rocks from the back of his truck and place them in the flower bed. At the time, I didn't realize at all how much that might possibly bless him. A few months later my mom and I were talking and she mentioned to me that her and my dad had been outside in the backyard and he became emotional. When he saw the rocks, he began to think about how hard I had worked to help him even under my physical circumstances. I think there're two main reasons I had the drive to accomplish that task. Number one, my dad has set a prime example of hard work and dedication over the years. He never stops until the job's done. He really instilled in me how to be strong, independent, and self-reliant, all while being honest and working as for the Lord and not man. Secondly, in my mind I wasn't limited to anything. I wasn't going to let something else (cancer or therapy) control what I could or couldn't do.

"Whatever you do, work at it with all your heart, as working for the Lord, not for human masters..."
Colossians 3;23

"Am I now trying to win the approval of human beings, or of God? Or am I trying to please people? If I were still trying to please people, I would not be a servant of Christ."
Galatians 1:10

Thursday, April 15th, 2010

You wanna know who frustrates me? Smokes, drinkers, and drug addicts frustrate me. Maybe it shouldn't bother me that other people make bad decisions for themselves because it is their body and their life and they can abuse it if they want to. But the reason it frustrates me so much is not because they are only making a bad choice, but because they actually have a choice and they aren't considering the outcome. Or maybe they are and they just don't care enough to let it slow them down. That's even worse. You see every person has the option to put harmful substances in their body that increase the chance of deadly diseases and ultimately death. Every person has the option to refrain from placing hazardous chemicals into their system. Well, everyone besides someone who accidently got a deadly disease from doing absolutely nothing wrong and now they have to place harmful chemicals into their system in order to stay alive, even though the long term side effects are much like those that would come from a life full of smoking, drinking, or drugs. Someone like the little toddler who knew no other way of living life other than feeling yucky a lot of the time because he had been going for treatments three years in a row since the age of two. Someone like the little girl in elementary school who probably wanted to curl her hair on Easter Sunday but this year she couldn't because those chemicals took all her hair away. Or, maybe someone like me who may not be able to go to a simple sleepover because being around a lot of people while staying up all night with no sleep can be dangerous for your health directly after being on chemotherapy. You see people are finding out every day they're fighting for their lives and at the exact same time people who have the potential to lead perfectly healthy lives are throwing it away. Babies, children, teenagers, mommy's, daddy's, grandmas and grandpas, brothers and sisters, cousins and friends, all those diagnosed we don't have a choice. It's inject the chemicals into our body or allow the deadly illness to spread and take over our body and eventually take our life. But the rest of you, you have a choice. So don't abuse it. No one wakes up one day and says to themselves "I think I'm going to be an alcoholic today." You never know which drink is going to push you over the edge to addiction, cause you to end your life or someone else's because of drunk driving, or give you liver cancer years down the road. Trying one cigarette may "relax" you, but at the same time it's destroying your heart and lungs. Not to mention the physical aging it does to your skin and teeth. And don't ever turn to drugs to escape from what you feel like you can't handle anymore. It just creates a completely different realm of new problems. Don't be one of the people who frustrate me, and if you already are then please take the time to consider what you're doing. You're slowly taking your own life. At least you have the power to control what's taking yours. Some people don't.

"But just as he who called you is holy, so be holy in all you do; for it is written: 'Be holy, because I am holy.'"
1 Peter 1:15-16

"'I have the right to do anything,' you say—but not everything is beneficial. 'I have the right to do anything'—but I will not be mastered by anything."
1 Corinthians 6:12

"Do you not know that your bodies are temples of the Holy Spirit, who is in you, whom you have received from God? You are not your own; you were bought at a price. Therefore honor God with your bodies."

1 Corinthians 6:19-20

In some ways cancer reminds me of baseball. A huge part of winning has to do with what's in your head. I heard someone say once that baseball was 90% mental and 10% physical. Maybe it's slightly different for beating cancer, but it still has a lot to do with what goes on in your head. If you step up to the plate and you're too afraid to swing, you have a 100% chance of not winning. If you tell yourself you are capable of defeating your opponent, you'll believe it and eventually live out that belief. One important thing to remember about baseball is never go down not swinging. One important thing to remember about cancer is never go down not fighting.

The one thing for me that feels just as good as knowing I'm fighting cancer and I'm winning is knowing that just by me simply living my life right now I'm changing and inspiring more people that I'll probably ever know. That's a life goal of mine that will never change.

"In the same way, let your light shine before others, that they may see your good deeds and glorify your Father in heaven."

Matthew 5:16

BIGGER

"I know that Jesus has the answer and he's way bigger than the cancer in you..."

- Hawk Nelson

Wednesday, April 21st, 2010

I wrote this on Monday night. For the past month or so, I haven't really slept on Monday nights. Even if I was just going in to get labs drawn the next day, the anxiety would keep me from getting much sleep. It got to the point where on Tuesday mornings before I would leave for the hospital I'd have to take a pill for nausea because it was so much on me. I couldn't enter CHKD without feeling like I was going to throw up. The smell of that Starbucks kills me. The smell of rubber gloves kills me. Certain words that I hear make me start gagging. But I don't have to deal with that anymore.

Tonight is the happiest night of my life. It's the night before my last chemo treatment. It may seem a little weird that the happiest night of my life is one that's just a few hours shy of chemotherapy, a word that makes me cringe, but it's true. When I was in the bathroom getting ready for bed, I had this feeling in my gut that I was just going to lay in bed tonight and cry, but not for the reasons most likely suspected. And I did.

When I laid down and closed my eyes I instantly pictured myself sitting on the bed in the E.R. with my parents across the room and the doctor close by with all six eyes staring me down waiting for my reaction and watching the tears start coming down as my world did too. Those words that the doctor had just said were beginning to sink into my mind and tear my world into tiny little bits and pieces. Those tears that I cried that night were streaming down my cheeks for a second time. Only this time, there was a drop of joy in each one. Because I had a slide show in my mind of everything I've been through, how far I've come, who I was on that hospital bed, and who I am now. I don't think I've ever had a more grateful moment in my life. I've never been more thankful than right now when I'm able to tell myself there's only one more to go and then that's it for what I pray will be forever. I've never been more thankful than right now when I can reflect on how I was given a second chance at life. It amazes me how that just three short months ago I have come this far. In three months I have been diagnosed with cancer, fought cancer, and nearly beat cancer. I have been to the lowest of lows, climbed every mountain possible, and now reached the highest of heights.

Before I laid in bed I looked at myself in the mirror and thought about all the hair I've lost. I thought about how humbling it was for me as a teenage girl to loose almost all of my hair. I want to say with everything in me that no teenage girl deserves that, because as you can imagine it can be devastating. However, there's a piece of me that feels maybe each and every teenage girl should feel just an ounce of what it feels like. Maybe then they wouldn't take things for granted or complain as much. I'm not saying that because I wish pain upon anyone, in fact I'm saying it for the complete opposite reason; because to me this has been the greatest experience of my life. Not necessarily the most enjoyable, but the one that has meant the most to me. And I'm honored, privileged, and humbled to be able to go through and share this with everyone.

I wouldn't take back that night in the E.R. for anything in the world. I wouldn't wish that the one bad cell inside of me that reproduced multiple times to form the tumor never existed. I wouldn't skip any step of this journey to get to the end faster no matter how much pain it caused. Those are things that broke me so I could be rebuilt. There is so much emotion inside of me right now I can barely feel anything at all. It's like I'm numb from the overwhelming amount of sensation. There's pain, anxiety, relief, joy, accomplishment, pride, humbleness, gratefulness, loneliness (because no one who hasn't gone through this can really and truly understand), togetherness, love, remembrance, hope, and victory. I feel like I'm giving an inadequate representation of the raw emotion I'm feeling, but the truth is, no words could ever possibly measure up. No matter how long or descriptive I write, you will never be able to sincerely understand the depth and perception of this story until you are the main character. Sometimes my heart and mind pay a bigger price for this than my body. But it's okay, because tonight is the happiest night of my life thus far.

Looking back at this now after typing it Monday night, it's even more of a relief. I wasn't going to add on to this because it's already extremely long, but I really felt like I should. As I was typing one of the last sentences, "Sometimes my heart and mind pay a bigger price for this than my body", I couldn't help but picture Jesus dying on the cross and what must have been going through his mind. I also went back to my first day in the hospital and telling my mom in my faint, helpless, voice, "You know mom, I just hope more people than just myself are changed from all of this." As I put everything together I was thinking about how Jesus must have felt something similar. Not that I'm even comparable with Jesus, I'm not saying that at all. He was a perfect, flawless, sacrifice. I am merely an imperfect mortal in dire need of that sacrifice. However, I bet our thoughts were somewhat related.

I bet as Jesus hung there dying, he must have been picturing all the people he was dying for who weren't going to be saved. I bet his head hurt worse from that than the crown of thorns piercing his brow. I bet his heart wrenched as he pictured his creation being eternally separated from

him all because they wouldn't accept what he had to offer.
I bet his heart hurt worse from that than the struggle to
catch every breath. I bet his heart and mind were paying a
much bigger price for all of that than his body. I bet Jesus'
whole story of death and resurrection changed the person
he was. I bet Jesus hoped and prayed with everything in
him that his story would change more people than just
himself. Just like me.

"Then Jesus said, 'Did I not tell you that if you believe, you
will see the glory of God?'"
John 11:40

"It is better to suffer for doing good than for doing wrong
if that is what God wants. Christ himself suffered for sins
once. He was not guilty, but he suffered for those who are
guilty to bring you to God. His body was killed, but he
was made alive in the spirit."
1 Peter 3:17-18

Radiation

When I finished my chemo treatment I thought my journey was coming to a close end. I felt somewhat like it was already completed, as opposed to simply in the home stretch. I don't think I quite realized how difficult the process of radiation is. For me, it seems it took more time to actually prepare me for receiving the treatment than my actual treatment period. I didn't suffer much from the short term side effects of radiation, just a sore throat and a little bit of energy loss. Sometimes, it would feel like the inside of my chest was sun burnt, like heart burn. My teeth became slightly sensitive as well, but it was nothing compared to chemo. Chemo took all of my hair whereas radiation just took a small section. The hardest part of it all was getting the pictures done so they could make the blocks. The blocks were more than mandatory because they prevented radiation from hitting anything that wasn't supposed to be treated, such as my heart and lungs. The process of making the blocks took much, much, longer than they originally planned and was a lot more painful than expected by anyone. My neck has a bruise from the piece of plastic they used to keep my head up. Before they switched my position my arms would go numb and uncontrollable from being placed above my head for so long. They had to make a plastic mask molded to the shape of my face used to pin my head back to the table to prevent it from moving (talk about claustrophobic). They used a blue marker to place x's on all of the targeted spots they would be hitting and covered them in this saran wrap type material. I had to be extremely cautious not to let the x's wipe off, which was intensely difficult between sweating, swimming, and showering in June. This may not make much sense, but radiation began to have a certain smell and taste. To this day I can still sense it when I get CAT scans.

"'In the same way I will not cause pain without allowing something new to be born,' says the Lord…"
                                    Isaiah 66:9

Last night as I was saying my prayers, I found them quite different than what your average sixteen year old girl has to pray for. When I was done, my eyes began to well up with tears. "Dear God, please help the men adding on to our house to get done soon. And please also help me to get my driver's license before my birthday. And dear Jesus, please, please, please, I pray with all of my heart that my scan will come out clear on Tuesday when I go to the hospital. Please, Lord Jesus. In your most glorious, powerful, beautiful, name I pray, Amen."

"Humble yourselves, therefore, under God's mighty hand, that he may lift you up in due time. Cast all your anxiety on him because he cares for you."

1 Peter 5:6-8

Facebook Status July 1st, 2010

Alexis Judy is thinking about how in 16 days I won't be 16 anymore. I think people kind of have this high expectation for the number 16. Almost like it's supposed to be the best year of your life or something. I don't really understand why though. If you ask me, life just keeps getting better and better as it goes on.

My favorite Bible verse has always been Hebrews 11:1, "Now faith is confidence in what we hope for and assurance about what we do not see." I love it because the reason God doesn't physically show himself or give us all the answers is because he wants us to have faith and believe. He wants us to have hope and confidence even though we can't physically see the outcome during our trials. It's not hard to have faith when you know what's going to happen, that's why by not knowing it requires trust. This will end up either leaving you hopeless for not doing so or feeling more empowered and in love with God than ever before.

This verse is to me the Biblical definition of the word "faith". It's very clear. Faith is having confidence in whatever it is you're hoping for, and being assured of things (like God or happy endings) even though right now you can't see them. After I actually lived this out, it took on a whole new meaning. I could literally feel a change in the way the words affected me. I not only understood what they meant, I felt it. Faith isn't just something that's meant to be understood by the mind, it's meant to be felt by the heart and lived out through our lives. I had confidence in my hope for the end of my cancer and to be eternally cured, and I was assured even though I couldn't see it happening that it would all come to an end because I had faith. Faith is not just a word that you have to stand for, there's a meaning behind it that we're all called to live out.

"In the same way, faith by itself, if it is not accompanied by action, is dead."

James 2:17

To make someone's day better just by smiling at them, that's a huge accomplishment. Who knows how far that frown would've driven them and who knows how far that smile will take them? You never know how far one gesture of love may go. It may reach farther than what your eyes can see or your ears can hear. You may live your whole life and never know. But don't choose not to do something just because you may never witness the affects.

"The King will reply, 'Truly I tell you, whatever you did for one of the least of these brothers and sisters of mine, you did for me.'"

Matthew 25:40

July 12th, 2010

A few days ago I was at a Casting Crowns concert and they started playing "Praise You In This Storm". As I began to sing the words and let them sink into my heart, my eyes began to well up with tears. Whenever I hear that song, I'm taken back to the moments I spent singing it lying in bed after having a chemo treatment. I would just repeat the chorus over and over again, "And I'll praise You in this storm, and I will lift my hands. For You are who You are, no matter where I am. And every tear I've cried, You hold in Your hand. You never left my side and though my heart is torn, I will praise You in this storm." As I was fighting back my tears, I had to stop singing. It was so overwhelming to sing those words after having made it through the storm and feeling the truth behind each statement. I will praise you no matter what's going on, even if there's no apparent reason. You are You, and You never change even though everything else will. Every tear I've cried, you value and treasure so much you hold it close to you forever as you dry them. My heart may be torn and broken and numb, but you still deserve my praise and allowing you to mend it is the only treatment for total healing. Crying while singing that song as it defined my life and then after as it was a "Thank you", was so empowering.

It's September now. The length between my writings gets greater and greater as time goes on. A lot has happened in the last three months. I had my once in a lifetime golden birthday, went on the greatest vacation ever, started teaching piano lessons, began my last year in high school. The list goes on and on but those are the biggest things. Today I went in for a follow up CT scan. I wasn't nervous because I trusted God and His promise to me. I wasn't naturally so calm, however, my God is supernatural and He works wonders.

"Not that we are competent in ourselves to claim anything for ourselves, but our competence comes from God."
2 Corinthians 3:5

Wednesday, September 1st, 2010

Summer 2010; So This Is How It All Went Down

Right now I'm thinking back to the month of May, back to the pre-summer days. I'm thinking back to when everyone was promising to make this the best summer of their lives. I'm remembering all the dreams and plans I had bottled up in my mind just ready to explode as I made them come true. I'm remembering the oath to myself to take risks, and live like every opportunity's your last because it very well could be. I'm reminiscing on who I was then, and who I am now. I'm reminiscing on how in some ways my summer was so different than I thought it would be, and how in some ways it was even better than I imagined.

This summer I:

- Got it started in Paradise! Went to Florida.
- Visited Disney World, Magic Kingdom, Epcot, Universal

Studios, Islands of Adventure, and Sea World. All in six days.

- Went to the best concert ever, Taylor Swift.

- Went to 3 days of concerts at Kings Dominion, with the best family members in the world. Seeing bands like Toby Mac, Skillet, Family Force Five, Brandon Heath, Chris Tomlin, Tenth Avenue North, and Casting Crowns.

- Almost blacked out for the first time on Dominator.

- Said good-bye to my sixteenth year of life, and hello to new beginnings.

- Had the most beautiful birthday party with the most beautiful people.

- Went to a family reunion. That's pretty big since it's only the second one in my lifetime.

- Broke my record for going to the most states in the least amount of time. In less than four months I went to; Florida, Georgia, South Carolina, North Carolina, Virginia, West Virginia, Ohio, Maryland, Indiana and Kentucky.

- Established the career path I'll be on for the rest of my life.

- Lost someone who was closest to me because they decided it just wasn't working for them anymore.

- Learned that I'll be okay because every time you lose something you gain something.

- Witnessed what it's really like to live two separate lives.

- Had my faith questioned and confirmed.

- Became thankful I know who I am, what I stand for, and what I believe; because what you stand for and what you believe make you who you are.

- Was away from home a lot, and even though my family was with me, I discovered there really is no place like home.

- Had a nightmare my parents divorced and woke up in the middle of the night crying. When I told my mom she said, "Now you know why it's so important that you marry the right person, why that's the biggest decision of your life other than being saved." I've never known anything other than that, but

-For the first time in my life I was scared to get married. She also pointed out the reason I had the nightmare is probably because so many people in our circle are having serious marriage problems. My parents definitely aren't, but so many people are. So in result, I

- Became much more aware that I'll never be satisfied if I have anything less than the relationship my parents have with each other.

- Took a ride in a Corvette.

- Went para-sailing.

- Rode on the back of a Harley.

- Saw the Jonas Brothers live for third time and proudly screamed loudly as if it was the first.

- Watched Demi Lovato preform live for the second time, and enjoyed it much more than the first time.

- Bought my last backpack.

- Took Senior pictures.

- Went swimming almost every day.

- Went boogie boarding.

- Learned how to skim board.

- Didn't have my camera because it was under repair, and it was awful.

- Went to the Creation Museum.

- Discovered that I actually like myself with really short hair, even though I never would have branched that far out had it been an option.

- Was told I look like Pink by more people than I can count on my hands and feet.

- Got a pet pig.

- Collected the first eggs from our chickens.

- Had my picture taken with a baby tiger in my lap.

- Had my picture taken with a monkey in my lap.

- Had surgery the day before my party.

- Met new people.

- Got lost in a HUGE maze.

- Survived many, many, hours in the car on road trips.

- Road the inter-tube and got slapped in the face with a fish for the first time. True story.

- Road a banana boat for the first time.

- Watched fireworks.

- Went to a baseball game. (What is a summer without at least one baseball game?)

- Saw a shark at the beach for the first time. Twice.

- Saw dolphins chase away sharks at the beach for the first time.

- Bought my senior prom dress.

- Prepared for my best friend to leave the country for seven months.

- Went to the biggest Zoo in the United States.

- Visited The Dixie Stampede, The Carolina Opry, The Alabama Theater, and Ripley's Aquarium.

- Went fishing.

- Went camping.

- Learned a lot.

- Experienced a lot.
- Loved a lot.
- Lost a lot.
- Gained a lot.
- Grew a lot.
- Enjoyed myself. A lot.

So, now, as I embrace the first week of my senior year in high school, I'll burn in my mind the passion I have at this moment to do the best I can. Everybody is inspired to do their absolute best the first week of school, maybe even the second, possibly even the third. But by the end of the first month it all dwindles down to nothing. You're not writing on the first few pages of your notebooks anymore, so the handwriting doesn't have to be perfect. Suddenly keeping your binders organized and your back pack cleaned out isn't so appealing. All the reading you were doing becomes dull and tiresome. Waking up early after staying up all night studying and finishing homework gets super old. And all the motivation you had to study and do your best to fully apply yourself disappears. I did my best to make this summer the best one I've ever had, and though it's a rather bold statement I think I would go so far c

it was. So, now, I'm going to go so far as to say

be the best year of school I've ever had. It is what I make it,

and I will make it the best.

"But seek first his kingdom and his righteousness, and

all these things will be given to you as well."

Matthew 6:33

"'For I know the plans I have for you,' declares the Lord,

'plans to prosper you and not to harm you, plans to give

you hope and a future.'"

Jeremiah 29:11

September 22nd, 2010

You said whoever loves you

You will save

Well I love you and I need

Strength to be brave

*Cause they tell me all these different things

But they don't know who You are

They tell me that I might not make it

But they don't know my heart

They wonder how I believe

And I wonder how they can't

How can life be worth living if you don't believe

you can?*

You said you'll protect those

Who know You

Well I know you and now

I know I'm safe

You said when I call you

You'll answer

Well I'm calling now to hear what you will say

* *

You said when I'm in trouble

You're by my side

That you'll rescue

And give me life

You said I will see how You can save

Well I see You in everything

And I've seen how You can save

* *

Life is only worth living when we believe we can.

Thanksgiving 2010

This year, I'm thankful for something that's never really even crossed my mind before. I'm thankful to be alive. I remember last year after dinner my aunt mentioned how skinny I looked, like I had lost weight. I recall how sick I felt and how sick I was. Little did we know. I hugged my mom on the way out the door to my cousin's house and she said, "Don't make me cry." I responded asking, "Why?", even though I already knew. She replied with, "Reminding me where we were at this point last year." I guess she didn't realize those same thoughts had been haunting me all day.

Black Friday 2010

This day last year I vividly remember. I remember waking up with no energy and feeling lifeless the whole day. I see myself reclined in the passenger's side of our Ford Excursion trying to sleep but not being able to because I had to keep coughing. I remember the feeling in my throat of not being able to hold back. I remember the feeling in my chest trying to fill my struggling lungs with oxygen. I was indeed almost lifeless. I hear Christmas carols playing on the radio, as I have flashbacks to my thoughts; wishing that my mom would hurry so we could go home. This year, I thought about that frequently. I felt and compared the difference between life and death; physically, spiritually, and emotionally.

So, it's the first week of December, almost a year since I was diagnosed. For the first time since then I have a cold. For the first time ever, that's almost petrifying. To hear myself cough, to not be able to control it, to taste cough drops, to have limited breathing, for my chest and throat to be sore, that's scary. I prayed one night that God would protect me in my sleep because even though I couldn't bring myself to admit it, I was scared of dying. I told my parents at dinner the other night that having a cold was scary. When they asked why I said, "Because the last time I had one I almost died." I'm not sure I'll ever be able to have a cold without psychotic fear again. Maybe I will, or maybe I won't. But for now, colds are related to diagnosis.

It's almost been one year. Time waits for no one. I am just now being hit with the reality that I've lived in since last January. I'm just now feeling it. It happened so fast I never stopped to try and believe it was actually happening. The pain was far too great to take on if I were to accept reality for what it was. I wasn't given a chance to feel, so I didn't ask for one. My emotions numbed themselves to prevent a breakdown. But now they're slowly beginning to feel again even though things are a little tingly. My senses are trying to adjust to the changes that were made when I was made senseless. It's unexplainable really. Like waking up from a dream and saying, "But wait, that really happened." It's almost like my body and mind put up a defense system and now they know that those events are far enough in the past that I can finally be introduced to them. Or maybe I'm just being forced to meet them as the time of year that they occurred draws near. All I know is life doesn't wait for you to get strong before it gives you battles. Time waits for no one. Life goes on.

"**There is a time for everything**, and a season for every activity under the heavens: a time to be born and a time to die, a time to plant and a time to uproot, a time to kill and a time to heal, a time to tear down and a time to build, a time to weep and a time to laugh, a time to mourn and a time to dance....**a time to tear and a time to mend**,...."

Ecclesiastes 3:1-7

Sometimes in life people get so caught up in winning the big battles they don't take the time to praise God for the victories over the small ones. For me, getting through

:mo was a battle, but a very small one compared to ιy body was facing fighting the cancer. I always prayed for God's help and thanked him for who He was and what He was doing during those little battles. Because I won the little battles, I ultimately won the big one. Being cancer free. See, once people overcome a huge obstacle in their life they praise God. But most of the journey along the way they forget to. Without victory over all of the small battles, you would never make it to the big ones. Stop and thank God for all of the little things He's helped you fight through. Thank him for getting you to where you are.

"I thank Christ Jesus our Lord, who has given me strength, that he considered me trustworthy, appointing me to his service."

1 Timothy 1:12

Because this is a sin cursed world, we almost always face a battle of some sort. Some much more serious than others. It is so important to praise God as you're heading into a battle. God doesn't particularly give us the battles that we face, but He does give us our victories. I remember the very first thing I said in my mind when I was dia...

"God, I can't do this by myself. I'm willing to fic

only if you're willing to help me." And that was it. Into

my battle I went.

"For the Lord your God is the one who goes with you to

fight for you against your enemies to give you victory."

Deuteronomy 20:4

"For the Lord takes delight in his people; he crowns the

humble with victory."

Psalms 149:4

"Where, O death, is your victory? Where, O death, is your

sting? But thanks be to God! He gives us the victory

through our Lord Jesus Christ."

1 Corinthians 15:55, 57

God didn't give me cancer. It wasn't a punishment

for some deep, dark, awful, secret sin I've been hiding for

years. Or any particular sin at all for that matter. It was

simply the result of being a mortal in a sin struck world.

A lot of people, even my closest Christian friends have

questioned why God would allow something like this to happen to someone who hasn't done anything to deserve it. If my God is a loving God, then why do people get cancer? Why do some children not have parents? Why do some people turn to drugs and alcohol? The truth of the matter is, we all forget what we truly deserve. Death. Jesus Christ conquered death so we could have the hope of living forever, but none the less, we're not in heaven yet. This world is full of sickness, disease, hurt, abandonment, addiction, and all other types of sin derived punishments. As a society, we tend to shift the blame. "Well, if God is in control, then why isn't he doing anything about it?" When man betrayed God and made the choice to sin in order to fulfill his fleshly desires, he fell short of the glory of God. He was no longer perfect and neither was the world around him.

"Neither this man nor his parents sinned," said Jesus, "but this happened so that the works of God might be displayed in him."

John 9:3

As sin entered the world, shame took over the heart of Adam and Eve. They realized what they had done. The Bible says for the first time directly after that moment, they were embarrassed to be walking around naked. Would you be embarrassed if your heart was naked and bare before God? Would you be ashamed if He could read your thoughts? Well, He can and He does. He wants nothing more than for you to reveal yourself to Him so He can reveal himself to you. Every day we fall so incredibly short of His glory. Yet, He pours out his forgiveness and mercy. God is holding the world in his hands. Certainly He could take control of your situation if you would give it to Him. God is a gentlemen and He is not going to take something you haven't given Him. Or, maybe you have given it to Him but it still seems like things are going all wrong. Remember that whatever it was you gave to him was his in the first place, and He has a specific purpose behind everything whether you can see it or not. If you begin your fight knowing the power of God and praising Him because of it, He will show up again. Do not be defined by the things going on in your life; be defined by God and the things He's going to use your life for.

"Not only so, but we also glory in our sufferings, because we know that suffering produces perseverance; perseverance, character; and character, hope. And hope does not put us to shame, because God's love has been poured out into our hearts through the Holy Spirit, who has been given to us."

Romans 5:3-5

"Rejoice always, pray continually, give thanks in all circumstances; for this is God's will for you in Christ Jesus."

1 Thessalonians 5:16-18

"He has made everything beautiful in its time. He has also set eternity in the human heart; yet no one can fathom what God has done from beginning to end. I know that there is nothing better for people than to be happy and to do good while they live."

Ecclesiastes 3:11-12

Don't ask God why you have certain trials, ask Him what He wants you to learn from them and how he wants to use you. Even though God's plan can be much different than our own, and often times much harder, it is so much more rewarding. I would have never chosen to go through cancer, but I wouldn't change that experience for anything. In order to grow in life we must experience different things. Some of those things are painful, but without experiencing them we wouldn't be able to change and become the people God wants us to be. I've also found that most of the time when you're going through a challenging situation, there's often someone a little bit behind you who's about to encounter the same thing or something similar. If the only reason I battled cancer was so that someone else believed they could battle whatever they're facing too, then that's a good enough reason for me.

"But he said to me, 'My grace is sufficient for you, for my power is made perfect in weakness.' Therefore I will boast all the more gladly about my weaknesses, so that Christ's power may rest on me. That is why, for Christ's sake, I delight in weaknesses, in insults, in hardships, in persecutions, in difficulties. For when I am weak, then I am strong."

2 Corinthians 12:9-10

"However, as it is written: 'What no eye has seen, what no ear has heard, and what no human mind has conceived' — the things God has prepared for those who love him".

1 Corinthians 2:9

I never saw myself fighting cancer. I never heard that one day I would have to fight for my life. I never imagined that God would draw near to me, change me, and use me to light the world in bigger ways than I knew were possible as a result of overcoming. And to think He prepared all of that just because I loved Him.

God is genuine and pure. His word is honest and He will always pull through for you if you believe that He is capable. Read His word and study His character and know that He is exactly who He says He is and He will do whatever He has promised. I think a lot of people these days, specifically the younger generations and people my age, look at the Bible as a book of the past. Even Christians who believe the Bible don't really take it in for all that it's worth. We, as Christians, need to realize that the Bible is very much alive. It's not just a book containing stories of old. It possesses a power to give us supernatural strength, encouragement, and direction to make it through life because it is the very word of God. We get frustrated when we feel like we can't hear God speaking to us but at the same time we aren't even applying what He said thousands of years ago to our lives. Often times it's so easy for us to run to people instead of God because we get an immediate response and there's also the physical presence. What we fail to realize is by reading God's word we will always receive a response. It may not be immediate, and it may not be the answer we're looking for, but there will be an answer. There will also be an abundance of promises that give us hope even when there's no logical reason to stay positive.

God loves you so much and wants nothing but the best for you. It's amazing to me that no matter where I'm at in life, God accepts me. When I'm in my weakest moment; in my most disgusting, repulsive, sinful, wretched state, completely breaking his heart, He loves me. Not only that, but when I'm doing good and everything's going right, when I'm in the word every day, talking to him all the time, and have peace that I'm in his will, He doesn't love me anymore than he does when I'm absolutely failing Him. God's love is so flawless it doesn't have the ability to elevate or decline based on our actions. Can you imagine where we would be if Christ stopped loving us when we failed him? Yet he knows that's when we need His love the most. When we're broken down to nothing, humbled beyond all reason because we see ourselves for who we really are, and when we're tormented by shame and regret, those are the moments when the precious love of Christ steps in to heal. Those moments when we realize we have nothing, we are nothing, and we can accomplish nothing without that kind of love in our lives.

Jesus, being the gentlemen that He is, will not show up uninvited. He wants to captivate you and form a beautiful relationship full of understanding and trust. Remember that it goes against the nature of God to try and shove something down someone's throat. If someone is saying something just to please you, then in their heart they don't really feel that way. That's why God gave us a choice. He wants us to choose to love Him by trusting, not because we have to. That's not true love. The first way we make the choice to trust God is by asking Him to come into our heart and save us. We're confessing that we're a sinner in dire need of a Savior, and we believe that Jesus died to wipe away our sins and save us from the eternal punishment we deserve because of that sin. Not only that, but he rose again three days later to return to heaven and prepare a place for us to stay with him for all of eternity. And someday, he's coming back. It's amazing how one step of faith in telling Jesus that you trust Him can radically change your world. That first step of faith made as a child ended up holding me together as a teenager and even now as a young adult.

"Whoever confesses that Jesus is the Son of God has God living inside, and that person lives in God. And so we know the love that God has for us, and we trust that love."

1 John 4:15-16

Once you've made the choice to trust God, you have to keep consciously making that choice just like I had to. The first choice God ever gave led to the fall of mankind. Due to doubt and lack of trust after a few whispers from the father of lies, Eve fell into the trap of fear and temptation and altered the course of world history. In her own selfishness and thirst for power, she wanted to control the situation; disregarding the warning that God had given her. Because Eve didn't listen to God and pursued her own plan, all of mankind was cursed. It is absolutely crucial that we trust God and what He tells us. Fear and doubt only bring harm whereas trusting will bring peace and hope. In essence, when you don't trust God you're saying, "Man, I don't know this problem is so huge. I don't even know if God can handle this one." Fear is a sin. With fear it is impossible to please God. It is not possible to hold on to fear and trust God at the same time. You either make the choice to fear the unknown or make the choice to trust the known.

"Do not be anxious about anything, but in every situation, by prayer and petition, with thanksgiving, present your requests to God. And the peace of God, which transcends all understanding, will guard your hearts and your minds in Christ Jesus."

Philippians 4:6-7

"Trust in him at all times, you people; pour out your hearts to him, for God is our refuge."

Psalms 62:8

"May the God of hope fill you with all joy and peace as you trust in him, so that you may overflow with hope by the power of the Holy Spirit."

Romans 15:13

"I have told you these things, so that in me you may have peace. In this world you will have trouble. But take heart! I have overcome the world."

John 16:33

"The Lord is with me; I will not be afraid. What can mere mortals do to me?"

Psalms 118:6

"The Lord is my light and my salvation - whom shall I fear? The Lord is the stronghold of my life - of whom shall I be afraid?"

Psalms 27:1

"He protects our lives and does not let us be defeated."

Psalms 66:9

"Be strong and brave. Don't be afraid of them and don't be frightened, because the Lord your God will go with you. He will not leave you or forget you."

Deuteronomy 31:6

"Where God's love is, there is no fear, because God's perfect love drives out fear...love is not made perfect in the person who fears."

1 John 4:18

The only way you can fight cancer at sixteen and never at any point be afraid is by knowing God and standing strong on His promises. In order to know God we must study His word. If we are not daily reading God's word we'll not only be distant from Him and unable to hear from him, we'll be unfamiliar with his promises. This is an extremely dangerous place to be. Through reading my Bible, I gained supernatural strength, wisdom, peace, and insight into the heart of God. The majority of the lessons learned and truths I discovered were revealed to me through God's word. Not to mention the countless promises I relied on. I learned more about God while fighting cancer than some people will learn in a lifetime, a lot of that due to the fact that I was so dependent upon his word.

"That is why you need to **put on God's full armor.** Then on the day of evil **you will be able to stand strong.** And **when you have finished the whole fight, you will still be standing.** So **stand strong, with the belt of truth** tied around your waist and **the protection of right living** on your chest. On your feet wear the Good News of **peace to help you stand strong.** And also **use the shield of faith** with which you can stop all the burning arrows of the Evil One. **Accept God's salvation** as your helmet, and **take the sword of the Spirit, which is the word of God. Pray** in the Spirit at all times with all kinds of prayers, **asking for everything you need.** To do this **you must always be ready and never give up**. Always pray for all God's people."

Ephesians 6:13-18

In Matthew 7, Jesus shares a metaphor that exemplifies this truth in our lives. He tells the story of a foolish man who builds his house upon sand. When the storm came his house was completely destroyed. On the other hand, we have a wise man who builds his house on a firm foundation of rock. When the storm came, it wasn't devastating for this man because his house did not move. The same goes for us. When we put our hope and our faith in things or people in this world, we will always be let down; especially when the storms of life come and tear everything apart leaving us helpless. On the contrary, when our hope and faith are built upon the solid, firm, foundation of Jesus Christ, when the storms of life come we will still be standing strong all the way until the end. Jesus is my rock and my foundation, he is the reason that I did not fall into the trap of fear.

"The rain came down, the streams rose, and the winds blew and beat against that house; yet it did not fall, because it had its foundation on the rock."

Matthew 7:25

In everything in life, no matter how painful, unbearable, or even death-stricken it may seem, it can be transformed into something beautiful. God works to make sure that the people who love Him and who have been called by Him for His purpose are taken care of. He selflessly works for our good. We have done nothing to deserve life, acceptance, love, or grace. But yet more often than not we expect it. Sometimes, we even get mad when we feel it being taken away. Maybe you don't feel angry, maybe you feel scared or alone. Well, you should know that in everything, meaning even the most horrid situation possible, God is working for your good if you love him. And you have been called according to His purpose; the purpose of your very existence, the purpose of being like Jesus. Because I loved Him, I was called to his purpose, and he worked for my good right in the middle of the valley of the shadow of death; empowering the weak to make me LIVESTRONG.

"We know that in everything God works for the good of those who love him. They are the people he called, because that was his plan."

Romans 8:28

"In your lives you must think and act like Christ Jesus. Christ himself was like God in everything. But he did not think that being equal with God was something to be used for his own benefit."

Philippians 2:5-6

"Whoever says that he lives in God must live as Jesus lived."

1 John 2:6

"But in every way we show we are servants of God: in accepting many hard things, in troubles, in difficulties, and in great problems. We are beaten and thrown into prison. We meet those who become upset with us and start riots. We work hard, and sometimes we get no sleep or food. We show we are servants of God by our pure lives, our understanding, patience, and kindness, by the Holy Spirit, by true love, by speaking the truth, and by God's power. We use our right living to defend ourselves against everything. Some people honor us, but others blame us. Some people say evil things about us, but others say good things. Some people say we are liars, but we speak the truth. We are not known, but we are well known. We seem to be dying, but we continue to live. We are punished, but we are not killed. We have much sadness, but we are always rejoicing. We are poor, but we are making many people rich in faith. We have nothing, but really we have everything."

2 Corinthians 6:4-10

It's important to remember that once we classify ourselves as Christians, we are making the choice to follow Christ and represent him in everything we say and do. Our lives are a constant testimony; that's not something to be taken lightly. While I was sick, I had a lot of people watching me and observing how I handled the things that were thrown at me. What we don't realize is we all have people watching us every day, people we may not even know about. No matter who you are or what you do, the way you live says everything about what you believe. It's said that true dignity is defined by the choices we make when we think no one is watching. We must consciously make the effort to make sure that we are always spreading the hope and love of Jesus even when we're not speaking and we think no one is watching.

I had a revelation yesterday that moved mountains in my soul. I realized that it is not my responsibility to be strong for everyone around me, and that's exactly what I've spent the last year of my life doing. I was so afraid that if I showed fear they would allow themselves to fear too. I was not only struggling to keep my own head above water, I was struggling to make sure I didn't pull everyone down with me. Whatever you're going through don't feel like you have to be what holds it together all the time and prevents it from falling apart. God asks for your burdens so He can handle the things he knows you're not capable of. I don't understand why we bring these things on ourselves instead of just letting Him deal with it all. He wants to deal with it because He knows how to. I am learning the art of how to be still and know that He is God.

"He says, 'Be still, and know that I am God; I will be exalted among the nations, I will be exalted in the earth.'"

Psalms 46:10

"Praise be to the Lord, to God our Savior, who daily bears our burdens. Our God is a God who saves; from the Sovereign Lord comes escape from death."

Psalms 68:19-20

It is kind of scary to think that even if I had every human on the face of the planet pray for me if it wasn't God's will it wouldn't make a difference. It's a good thing I didn't think about this until after I had been through treatment. However, afterwards I then encountered the thought of relapse. What if it was a part of God's plan for me to relapse? First of all, God's will be done. Having said that, I do believe in the power of prayer. God says where two or more are gathered in His name, He is there with them. I believe that it moves the heart of God to see hundreds of His children come to him asking, some begging, on behalf of one specific child. The Bible says that the requests of His people influence Him. I know God has placed peace in my heart that even some Christians can't understand because it passes ALL understanding. See, this is where the faith aspect comes in. When everything in your life is fairly stable and you have little need for faith, it's quite easy to obtain it. But when everything in your life is unstable and you have little reason to have faith, that's when you need it the most. That's when your faith develops. If you have no reason to hold on to your faith, you're more likely to let it go whenever it's convenient. But when you realize that faith is the only reason for your existence and sometimes the only thing you have to hold onto, you begin living by it. Faith grows by being stretched. So, instead of waiting for a situation to arise where you will need your faith to make it through, realize that you need your faith to survive on a day to day basis.

"For where two or three gather in my name, there am I with them."

Matthew 18:20

"....If you do not stand firm in your faith, you will not stand at all."

Isaiah 7:9

Wednesday, March 9th, 2011

Today I feel inspired to write. I suppose this is because my emotions have been picked up and spun frantically around like the winds of a hurricane based on some unfortunate events that have happened to a few people in my life; and writing is just what I do when that happens.

Besides all of this, my day was absolutely fabulous on a personal note. Especially when I started talking to God and I remembered something; I remembered being in a situation where all I could do is pour my heart out. That is literally the only hope I had to hold onto. Hoping that God would choose to be proactive and heal me. And then I remembered how blessed I am because He chose to do so, and he really didn't have to. Every day as I lift up the people in my life who are battling cancer, or just battling life, I'm reminded of this. I remember that I was the closest to God when I needed Him the most. I remember that I need Him every day. I need Him to watch over me and protect me and keep me safe. I need him to give me wisdom and discernment to make the right choices. I need him to continue healing me because see, most people don't realize this, but I'm not even considered cancer free until I've had five years with clear scans. I need Him to search out my heart and make me a better person. I need Him to use all of the gifts and talents that He's given me however He needs them to be used. I need Him to constantly remind me of where I've been, where I'm at, and where I'm being taken. I need Him to stretch my faith because that's the only way it can grow. Even if it petrifies me, the more stretch the more growth. I need Him to remind me that my life is not about me.

"Live in harmony with one another. Do not be proud, but be willing to associate with people of low position. Do not be conceited."

Romans 12:16

"Do not withhold good from those to whom it is due, when it is in your power to act."

Proverbs 3:27

"Whoever tries to keep their life will lose it, and whoever loses their life will preserve it."

Luke 17:33

"So whether you eat or drink or whatever you do, do it all for the glory of God."

1 Corinthians 10:31

This world is full of evil. Hurt. Sickness. Depression. Death. Pain. Sadness. Fear. Deception. Lies. Hatred. Starvation. Slavery. Murder. Betrayal. Pain. War. Bullies. Sin. All on a physical and spiritual level. And in the midst of all of this, in the midst of fighting so hard day to day just to keep moving forward, there is one thing that never changes. Or more so, one person. God. He's the same all the time, no matter what's going on around us. His love doesn't elevate or decline. He is always right there, He never leaves. He is who He says He is and He does what He says He's going to do. Even if we can't see it, or we're too numb to feel. Faith isn't a feeling, it's a choice. It's not the overwhelming emotion we get when we're worshipping God, that's worship. It's not dying to self and meeting other people's need first, that's being a servant. It's not showing up at church every Sunday and answering questions in Sunday School, that's being dedicated to your religion. All of these things are factors that come from having faith; however, you can have all of these things and have very little faith. Only hardships can produce faith, because it's in our most difficult seasons that our faith is really put to use. When we're not in the midst of trials, we have little need for much faith. Faith is choosing to rely on God and fully trusting Him even though you can't see what's ahead. It's coming to a point where you give up total control and let God lead you. Faith is trusting what you can't see.

So, never complain about what's going on in your life no matter how bad it is, because there is always something way worse going on somewhere. Realize that whatever you're dealing with is an exercise to strengthen your faith. Trials produce perseverance, and perseverance, faith. I may have finished treatment, but I'm still battling the prevention of getting cancer again. But that's nothing compared to some peoples battles. I feel like I've posted 100

Facebook notes telling people to never complain, always have faith, and how unbelievably extraordinary God is; but then I realized that 100 wouldn't be enough.

"For those who are led by the Spirit of God are the children of God."

Romans 8:14

August 15th, 2011

    This morning in church my pictures started off the senior slideshow. I can't grasp this whole "Alumni" concept. It's still foreign to me. I could've done the whole cap and gown, walk down the aisle, make your speech, get your diploma, take your pictures so you can post them on Facebook thing; but I guess whatever desire I ever had to do that kind of faded away when my desire to finish high-school trumped everything. When I think about graduating high-school, I don't think about the last four years. I think about how I'm ending another chapter in my story. It seems to me like going from pre-school to kindergarten, through elementary school into middle school, and then drifting into high-school and somehow making your way all kind of blend together. Like paragraphs. They all have different points but they unite in order to tell one part of a story. But now, that part of the story is coming to a close. The little girl with the bouncy blonde curls and big blue eyes is walking headlong into a giant scary sea of grown up faces. Every scraped knee, every word I've ever wanted to take back, every memory I've wanted to fade away into nothingness, every moment I want to remember until I die, every accomplishment that's ever made me feel like I've actually done something worthwhile, it's all brought me to where I'm at right now.

I guess going through life is like watching a chick flick, even when the difficult part comes and you get that nervous feeling in your stomach when you just wanna scream, "JUST FIX IT ALREADY!", it's okay because you know everything turns out perfect in the end. That's how it is in life. You get to these points where you get that nervous feeling and you just wanna scream, but something keeps you holding on because you know if things aren't right then it's not the end.

Now it's the end of the summer, and this is more real than ever. I'm ready to scream. College plans aren't just something I tell people about and ponder every now and then, it's my life. It's almost like starting all over. There's no one to make sure you're getting your work done, because no one really cares. You do it or you don't, you pass or you fail, it's your future not theirs. You're not forced to see your friends all the time anymore and your all headed in totally different directions, so you find out who your true ones are. Whether you want to or not. Your parents can't take the blame anymore when you mess up, because you're responsible for yourself. No one tells you what you have to study or learn until you choose for yourself. You have to live with the choices that you make, and you have to make those choices for yourself regardless of what other people are going to think. You're choosing the path that's going to affect every day of the rest of your life. This is the last season where it's okay for everything to be about you. Once you get involved in a really serious relationship, get married, have kids. Everything changes. Priorities change. Needs change. You change. It's the last chance to accomplish things you can only accomplish before you have bigger commitments. I've been raised my whole life knowing these things and being prepared for them, but there's a difference between knowing something and feeling it. There's a difference between preparing for life and moving on in life.

It would be easier to stay the same and never change or move or grow. It would be challenging to hold on forever, but it would be less painful than letting go. It would feel more comfortable to stick with what I've always known, but it would be a lot less exciting than seeing God's plan unfold. There's a world to be changed and a love to reach souls, I have a future already planned for me, and I want to fulfill all God's goals. Even though this is the end of a chapter, it's the beginning of one crazy beautiful story. Hello world.

"Your beginnings will seem humble, so prosperous will your future be."

Job 8:7

Monday, December 12th, 2011

   So, I wrote this for English this past semester, and I figured that more people should read it than just my professor since the whole source of inspiration was childhood cancer awareness. I simply have one request before you exit this page and go back to your newsfeed: I don't want you to just read it, tell me what you think, or share it. Even though I'd be genuinely thankful for any of those. Really and most importantly, before you refresh your browser, I want you to refresh your outlook on life.

Memoir Of A Survivor   10/6/2011

   Who knew a day of the week could literally make your stomach turn. Tuesday. That was the day. The approach of Tuesday made me want to curl up into a ball and forget the world. See, every Tuesday I was forced to enter through two sliding glass doors into any child's worst nightmare. The sharp, distinct, over-powering, smell of Starbucks coffee that engulfed the front desk area attacked my senses. Even if I wasn't there to receive treatment, just the visual environment could paralyze my capability to feel normal, or maybe even to feel at all. Hearing the quick "ding!" of the elevator sent shockwaves through my body. It's amazing really, how a smell, a sight, a sound, has the power to overtake you. Even if I wasn't going to receive medicine that would make me vomit, I had to take medication to rid the nauseous feeling. Tuesday was the day I went to the hospital to receive chemotherapy.

After the quick "ding!" of the elevator, my mom and I would step inside and make our way up to the next floor. Exiting quickly, I was already thinking about how much I'd rather be anywhere but in this place. Making our way into the clinic waiting room, we would open the door to reveal either smiling children partnered by their parents, or vacancy. The amount of activity was dependent upon the level of chaos for that particular day. You wouldn't think in a place like that you'd see any smiling faces at all, but yet those are the happiest people I've ever seen in my life. Happiness comes from being content, and when you realize how precious life is and you become content with just simply having it, you really understand that you don't have anything to complain about. Walking through the door and over to the front desk on the left hand wall, my mom begins the signing in process. The ladies on the other side of the glass window grin dramatically, almost as if they were excited to see me every single time. I never quite understood why. Taking a seat in the waiting room, we'd watch as different children would enter and leave with their parents. Some with lots of hair, some with none. Some wearing hats, some wearing slippers and pajamas. Some pushing an IV, some being pushed in wheel chairs. Some dancing around restlessly anxious to leave, some standing tall even though they look like they could collapse at any given moment. Some happy, some upset. All wearing the faces of heroes.

Eventually, after a typically long period of waiting, a nurse would crack open the second door of the waiting room and call my name, "Alexis?" As I got up from my chair, they would say hello and ask me how I was doing.

It was a sharp right turn into the room where they take vitals, and every time it was the same procedure. The exact same questions in pretty much the exact same order, even if the nurse was different. "Last name? Date of birth? Any pain going on today?" Record blood pressure, height, and weight, and then draw blood. Drawing blood was always a battle. It was as if my veins knew exactly what was coming and as soon as the needle went in they'd run and hide. Once the blood was drawn, I knew that part of the day was over and my mom and I could head to the back part of the clinic. It was always just my mom and I because they're so picky about who they allow inside. With good intentions, of course. It's not optional to be cautious while your body's undergoing chemotherapy. Your immune system becomes so weak and defenseless. Frequently people have to be hospitalized because they aren't producing enough white blood cells. You see, chemo doesn't just kill the bad stuff in your body, it kills the good stuff too. As a result, I had to have shots every day to boost my immune system to prevent serious illness and hospitalization.

Once we arrived at the back of the clinic, we'd find two chairs beside each other and sit down. These chairs weren't normal chairs though. First of all, they had the appearance of over-sized dentist chairs. Placed right in the center of the room, almost as if they were the focal point, a teal-green color, and big too. The second reason they weren't normal chairs is because these chairs held small, innocent, clueless children just waiting for the drugs to enter their fragile little bodies. Some had an idea of what was coming and already felt sick, like me. I didn't have to wait for the medicine to enter my body before I wanted to throw up. Then there were the really small ones, like toddlers, who made hooking up the IV to their port a matching game with the nurses. If only they knew.

Day's at clinic were long and exhausting, especially every other week when I received chemo. At first, that was an all-day process. It would drag on and on miserably until I could finally go home just to lay in bed for the next few days. It presented more than just a physical battle, it was emotional, mental, and spiritual, too. It reminds me of my favorite movie, A Walk To Remember, when the teenage girl is fighting cancer herself and says, "I do not need a reason to be angry with God." Sometimes, even when I felt the weakest, I also felt the strongest.

The thing about cancer is it never leaves you. The disease itself may leave your body, but the remains of tattered memories are permanent. As they become more distant and vague, I find myself fighting to remember. The whole experience changed everything about who I am and how I live my life. For example, if I even begin complaining, an instant guilt takes residence deep within me because I remember that I have nothing to complain about. Thus, the disease is still affecting me even though it's no longer taking my life. I feel like a lot of people think that because I'm no longer physically battling cancer, it's no longer a battle for me. However, that is simply not true. Once someone is personally affected by cancer, the battle never ends. The whole purpose behind me sharing this story is to give a realistic view on how cancer affects people, specifically children. I chose this memory above everything else I've experienced in life because this situation affected and changed me the most. Now, I hope that my story can change other people as well.

"Surely the righteous will never be shaken;

they will be remembered forever."

Psalms 112:6

How will you be remembered?

Be love.

"Do everything in love."

1 Corinthians 16:12

"Dear friends, let us love one another, for love comes from God. Everyone who loves has been born of God and knows God. Whoever does not love does not know God, because God is love."

1 John 4:7-8

"I pray that out of his glorious riches he may strengthen you with power through his Spirit in your inner being, so that Christ may dwell in your hearts through faith. **And I pray that you, being rooted and established in love, may have power,** together with all the Lord's holy people, **to grasp how wide and long and high and deep is the love of Christ, and to know this love that surpasses knowledge** - that you may be filled to the measure of all the fullness of God."

Ephesians 3:17

"And over all these virtues put on love, which binds them all together in perfect unity."

Colossians 3:14

"Jesus replied: 'Love the Lord your God with all your heart and with all your soul and with all your mind.' This is the first and greatest commandment. And the second is like it: 'Love your neighbor as yourself.'"

Matthew 22:37-40

"If I speak in the tongues of men or of angels, but do not have love, I am only a resounding gong or a clanging cymbal. If I have the gift of prophecy and can fathom all mysteries and all knowledge, and if I have a faith that can move mountains, but do not have love, I am nothing. If I give all I possess to the poor and give over my body to hardship that I may boast, but do not have love, I gain nothing.

Love is patient, love is kind. It does not envy, it does not boast, it is not proud. It does not dishonor others, it is not self-seeking, it is not easily angered, it keeps no record of wrongs. Love does not delight in evil but rejoices with the truth. It always protects, always trusts, always hopes, always perseveres.

Love never fails. But where there are prophecies, they will cease; where there are tongues, they will be stilled; where there is knowledge, it will pass away. For we know in part and we prophesy in part, but when completeness comes, what is in part disappears. When I was a child, I talked like a child, I thought like a child, I reasoned like a child. When I became a man, I put the ways of childhood behind me. For now we see only a reflection as in a mirror; then we shall see face to face. Now I know in part; then I shall know fully, even as I am fully known.

And now these three remain: faith, hope and love. But the greatest of these is love."

1 Corinthians 13

Mission: To Literally Be Love

Alexis is patient, Alexis is kind. Alexis does not envy, Alexis does not boast, Alexis is not proud. Alexis does not dishonor others, Alexis is not self-seeking, Alexis is not easily angered, Alexis keeps no record of wrongs. Alexis does not delight in evil but rejoices with the truth. Alexis always protects, always trusts, always hopes, always perseveres.

"We love because God first loved us." 1 John 4:19

Tonight is January seventh, 2012.

Exactly two years ago tomorrow will be the date I went to the emergency room the night I was originally diagnosed.

I'm eighteen now.

I never imagined having this much life experience at eighteen.

I have been forever changed.

"Come and hear, all you who fear God; let me tell you what he has done for me."

Psalms 66:16

"Praise be to God, who has not rejected my prayer or withheld his love from me!"

Psalms 66:20

_____

_____

"Then Jesus said, 'Did I not tell you that if you believe, you will see the glory of God?'"

John 11:40

_____

_____

"Blessed is she who has believed that the Lord would fulfill his promises to her!"

Luke 1:45

_____

_____

_____

_____

_____

_____

_____

_____

_____

_____

I'd like to say thank you from the bottom of my heart for taking your time to read what I have to say. It truly means the world to me. Also, you should know that I've been praying for you for quite some time now. You're very, very, very, loved. Whether you realize and accept it or not. I very much hope this story impacted you the same way it impacted me. See, this isn't really a "book". This is just a journal. My journal. The one I published so that people could read it and relate to it and be "mutually encouraged" (Romans 1:12) by my faith. This isn't about me. This is about what God can do through His people if they love and trust Him enough. This is about legacy, my legacy, your legacy. A predestined legacy waiting to be fulfilled. What will your legacy say about you long after you no longer exist?

"However, as it is written: 'What no eye has seen, what no ear has heard, and what no human mind has conceived'- the things God has prepared for those who love him..."

1 Corinthians 2:9

"Rejoice in the Lord always. I will say it again: Rejoice! Let your gentleness be evident to all. The Lord is near. Do not be anxious about anything, but in every situation, by prayer and petition, with thanksgiving, present your requests to God. And the peace of God, which transcends all understanding, will guard your hearts and minds in Christ Jesus...Whatever you have learned or received or heard from me, or seen in me – put it into practice. And the God of peace will be with you...I know what it is to be in need, and I know what it is to have plenty. I have learned the secret of being content in any and every situation...I can do all things through him who gives me strength."

Philippians 4:4-13

"No, in all these things we are more than conquerors through him who loved us."

Romans 8:37

In August 2012, I had an interview with my local crisis pregnancy center. During that interview, I had to share my personal beliefs and convictions. I explained why my relationship with Christ has been so life changing and why it is the most precious thing I have. In fact, it's worth nothing compared to anything else. (Philippians 3:8) Nothing I ever accomplish or possess will compare to the greatness I have found in placing my trust in Jesus. Not only for the salvation he's given me, but for everything in life. At the end of the interview, one of the ladies looked at me, smiled, and said, "Christ illuminates from your pores." That is one of the absolute greatest compliments I have ever received and could ever ask for. I take it very seriously that my life is a constant testimony and I have a call to live a holy and righteous life pleasing to God, as does every other person claiming to be a Christian. This means always taking a stand for what's right. I would rather be hated for who I am than liked for someone I am not. I take very seriously the command to love by being love. Being a Christian doesn't only mean following Christ and obeying the rules of God's word; it means being the hands and feet of Christ and unleashing the power of the gospel. I don't want people to ask if I'm a Christian with a hint of skepticism. I want them to ask confident that they already know the answer I'll give them, only asking to confirm what they can already tell. It is a daily prayer that I may be completely transparent and the love of Christ would absolutely define me, my life, my words, and my actions, and radiate through me. And when people wonder what's different about me and my life, I'll be able to tell them all of the glorious things Jesus has done for me and through me and why I have hope. It is my prayer that by sharing my testimony of hope others will either come to know Christ or come to know him better than before. Not because I've done anything out of the ordinary, but because of Jesus; because he loves me, and because they realize how much he loves them too.

_____

_____

"...Always be ready to answer everyone who asks you to explain about the hope you have,"

     1 Peter 3:15 (NCV)

_____

_____

_____

_____

Special Thanks

Mom & Dad – I know there were moments when you probably thought I was insane for doing this and that you were insane for encouraging me to do it, but you were always there. You've never failed to set an example of genuine faith in God regardless of your circumstances, and I'm forever grateful for the faith you also had in me. Thank you.

Uncle Joe – I'm not sure if you're even slightly aware of this, but you've encouraged me so much. Every time we talk you're so interested and fascinated by whatever it is I'm doing in life. After one of our more recent conversations you said, "You're gonna make it." I haven't forgotten that. Thanks for passionately and whole-heartedly believing in me.

Irmie – You're always reiterating how proud you are of me and how much you love me. I just want you to know that I've never doubted that. Thank you for being such a huge part of my life and always assuring me that I can accomplish anything I set my mind to. It's humbling to be your "inspiration", and I'm honored.

Harrison – I'm so proud of you! Your spiritual maturity is far beyond your years and your creativity greater than you realize. Your convictions inspire me.

Hayden – You may be little, but your personality is so precious to me! You are constantly thinking of others. Not only are you self-motivated, but you are such a hard worker. We can all learn from you.

Caely – Thanks for always having my back. I need someone to be blunt with me, and you're really great with that. I can't think of many things that are greater than having a sister for a best friend.

Cameron & Cassidy – Ya'll are the greatest cousin-siblings anyone could ask for. You supported me so much throughout my treatment process. Cass, thanks for that sweet letter you wrote me even a few years after treatment before I went in for a follow-up scan. You understood how much I didn't wanna go to the hospital. Never lose your big heart and compassion for others.

Aunt JoAnne & Uncle Louis – Thank you for all of the prayers, encouragement, and support you've provided. From staying the night with my siblings the night I was admitted, to bringing me that white pizza in the hospital, to the ring before port surgery, to being excited over the first time I could put my hair back in a short little ponytail. These are moments I'll never forget.

Miss Diane – I just want to thank you for investing in me. In some moments you're tough because you have the ability to see my full potential but you're encouraging always because you know that's what propels me. You're truly one of the most influential people in my life and my musical career wouldn't be possible without you.

Allison – I'm sorry for all those times you had to hear about how Satan was putting negative thoughts in my head regarding this project, but I'm thankful that you were there with words of encouragement. Also, thank you for proofreading one of the first pitches and assuring me that there would actually be people interested in what I have to say. You're an awesome best friend.

LeahAnn – I want to thank you again for keeping a journal while I was going through treatment and then giving it to me. It was so fantastic to read my journey from someone else's perspective. Thank you for caring so much about me and encouraging me. You and your family have blessed me greatly. I'm thankful for our lifelong friendship and I'm excited for the future.

Ellie – Thank you for being there from the time I was in the hospital. Thank you for setting an example of what it's really like to rely on God for literally everything. It's true that friendship isn't about how long or how far apart you are, but about how you can be apart for a long time and nothing changes. You're fantastic.

Maw Maw – I wish you could've read this book before you went to meet Jesus. Then again, you totally got the point. When I get to heaven, you can introduce me to grandpa and we'll talk about it. Thank you for being one of the Godliest women I've ever known. Thank you for encouraging me to continue pursuing the piano, and for giving me that gift to inherit. Thank you for always providing cookies or sharing your chocolate. Thank you for leaving a legacy powerful enough to outlive your lifetime.

Everyone at Westbow Press – Thank you so much for believing in this project and for making it possible. Without you, my dreams would still be dreams instead of reality.

To every person who has ever prayed for, encouraged, and supported me along the way. There are far too many to name individually. To all the people who had never met me but sent me messages while I was sick, thank you. Because when someone who's never even met you cares enough to encourage you and tell you how your life is making an impact; that is often times more powerful than when those you love the most do so.

To every person who in any way implied to me that this book was a good idea, thank you. To every individual who believed in me, in this book, and in the work God could accomplish through both of us. Your thoughts, prayers, and support are much appreciated. You helped me maintain the confidence to rid the doubt. Thank you.

God, I feel like I've been walking with a blindfold on throughout this whole process yet you've not once failed in leading me. In your perfect way, in your perfect timing, you placed everything together. I couldn't see what was coming next, I still don't know what's coming next, but I knew what you were calling me to do and I still have this unwavering faith. Thank you for that. Thank you for being the author and perfecter of my faith. Thank you for never failing me. Thank you for always, always, always, loving me. Even when I don't deserve it.

Stay Connected

Facebook: www.facebook.com/AlexisJudyOfficial

Twitter: @LexiJudy07

YouTube: www.youtube.com/user/AlexisJudy

Instagram: LEXIJUDY

Pinterest: www.pinterest.com/AlexisJudy

Website: www.AlexisJudy.com

CPSIA information can be obtained at www.ICGtesting.com
Printed in the USA
LVOW13s1448300614

392345LV00001B/303/P